2

NEUROSCIENCE RESEARCH PROGRESS

FUNCTION AND METABOLISM OF AGING

LONGITUDINAL NEUROIMAGING EVALUATIONS

NEUROSCIENCE RESEARCH PROGRESS,

Additional books and e-books in this series can be found on Nova's website under the Series tab.

GERIATRICS GERONTOLOGY AND ELDERLY ISSUES

Additional books and e-books in this series can be found on Nova's website under the Series tab.

NEUROSCIENCE RESEARCH PROGRESS

FUNCTION AND METABOLISM OF AGING

LONGITUDINAL NEUROIMAGING EVALUATIONS

YONGXIA ZHOU

nova
Medicine & Health
New York

Library of Congress Cataloging-in-Publication Data

ISBN: 978-1-53615-613-3

Published by Nova Science Publishers, Inc. † New York

Contents

PREFACE

It is well known that maintaining brain functional active and metabolic equilibrium is important to a healthy brain and especially for people with age. For instance, cerebral blood flow (CBF) to cerebral metabolic rate of oxygen ($CMRO_2$) coupling decrement and cerebral metabolic rate of glucose (CMRglu) reduction had been observed at normal aging. However, several metabolic/cardiovascular risks increase with age as well, including insulin resistance increment possibly due to hypertension and disrupted glucose/insulin metabolism that were correlated with blood metabolites. Thus it is important to illustrate the dynamic profiles of blood flow, oxygen utilization (i.e., extraction) and glucose metabolism, lipid and oxidative metabolism both regionally and globally to better understand the underlying brain functions and physiology with aging. More detailed quantifications of pathological burdens with advanced molecular imaging techniques at normal aging and in neurodegenerative disorder including Alzheimer's disease (AD) will be described. Both baseline and longitudinal imaging analyses and correlations with neurocogntive tests as well as cardiovascular risk factors could provide distinct and confirmative perspectives relating to the pathophysiology of aging-related diseases such as dementia and diabetes.

The aim of this book is intended to provide both beginners and experts in biomedical imaging and health care a broad picture as well as new developments in brain function and metabolism of aging using innovative neuroimaging techniques and advanced longitudinal/ correlational analysis. Methods and data presented in this book with novel experimental designs and protocols, especially longitudinal investigation of multiple imaging metrics from microvascular, micro-structural to systematic functional, metabolic and neuropathological perspectives will help improving diagnosis and early prevention of common diseases at middle age such as metabolic syndrome and early dementia. Some promising prevention strategies such as arts therapy, aerobic exercise and calorie restriction will be introduced additionally with imaging evidence. Results presented will help improving diagnosis accuracy, staging and prediction, in addition to determining the phases and trajectories of disease progression with age, endothelial dysfunction and deficits in metabolic syndrome. Together with solid and complete imaging evidence, early detection and treatment could be achieved with the ultimate goal of improving quality of life at earlier age and extending longevity. This book would hopefully capture the interests of colleagues in fields of aging-related research, and could help convey the methodological developments of brain function and metabolism at normal aging as well as longitudinal changes.

Chapter 1 - Longitudinal studies can be used for causality inference based on the temporal orders and correlations among multiple parameters at different time points. Accounting for individual differences including demographic and biological factors is another advantage of longitudinal investigation that uses individual baseline and usually applies paired statistical examination between baseline and follow-ups for the same subject population. Early detection and prevention play a crucial role in treatment and improvement of brain health, and literatures related to longitudinal neuroimaging studies with age are limited. Furthermore, identifying longitudinal changes of neuroimaging parameters at short interval (for instances, 6 months to 72 months) could help determining disease phase (acute vs. chronic), quantifying trajectories of disease progression (early vs. late stage), and prediction of long-term aging-related effects with more complementary health profile. It is important to illustrate the dynamic profiles of blood flow, oxygen utilization (i.e., extraction fraction) as well as glucose, lipid and oxidative metabolism both regionally and globally to better understand the underlying brain functions and physiology with aging. For the past few years, multiple applications of the integrated PET/MRI imaging including inflammation, functional metabolism and microstructure mapping have been reported. The aim of this chapter is to review multi-modality neuroimaging technique and applications, as well as to introduce the main topics of this book- longitudinal imaging and applications in aging and dementia.

Chapter 2 - Revealing brain functional and micro-structural changes over a relatively short period at individual levels are especially important given that many risks associated with age including vascular -metabolism and neuroinflammation increases and could confound the baseline fMRI parametric images. Cellular-level axonal injury and/or demyelination as well as dispersed mesoscopic level substance abnormal aggregation and structural/functional abnormality could occur in short subacute/acute phases, while only a few studies reported literatures related to longitudinal changes with age are limited with only our previous fMRI findings. Longitudinal data were used to characterize these multiple parameters including random intercept and interval per individual. No significant age by gender interactions have been found to either diffusion tensor imaging (DTI) fractional anisotropy (FA) or diffusivity metrics. The interval effective regions showed longitudinal change of FA and radial diffusivity (RD)/axial diffusivity (AX) values remained similar to the aging results found with cross-sectional data. Significant correlations between DTI and fMRI metrics as well as between imaging and neurocognitive data including speed and memory were found. Our results indicate significant and consistent age, gender and apolipoprotein E (APOE) genotypic effects on structural and functional connectivities at both short-interval and cross-sectional ranges, together with correlational neurocognitive functions.

Chapter 3 – Our previous baseline results suggested that newly developed MRI biomarkers of endothelial dysfunction (EDF) were sensitive to both age and smoking effects that act independently and similarly. The purpose of this study is to assess various surrogates of EDF at 18-month follow-up compared to baseline in smokers and older subjects. Measures of peripheral vascular reactivity were assessed via dynamic venous susceptometry and oximetry, arterial velocimetry and multi-segment pulse-wave velocity (PWV) of thoracic and abdominal aorta in the form of an integrated protocol with a time-resolved multi-echo gradient-recalled echo (GRE) sequence. Total 113 subjects out of 169 baseline participants finished 18-month 2nd visits consisted of 39 young non-smokers, 14 young smokers, 30 old non-smokers and 30 old smokers. Vascular reactivity was evaluated following cuff-induced hyperemia via time-resolved blood flow velocity and venous saturation of oxygen (SvO_2) in the femoral artery and vein, respectively, by quantifying post-occlusion change relative to baseline values. Velocimetry-based arterial parameters included pulse ratio, hyperemic index and forward flow time. PWV was assessed in aortic arch, thoracoabdominal aorta and iliofemoral arteries. Two-way ANOVA indicated that there was no interaction between smoking and age ($P = 0.09\text{-}0.78$) for all parameters evaluated at follow-up visits. Paired t-test for the same MRI parameter between two visits across all subjects showed significant longitudinal worsening in several parameters including reduced overshoot ($P = 0.003$) and arterial hyperemic index ($P < 0.0001$), as well as increased pulse ratio ($P < 0.0001$) and iliofemoral PWV (ifPWV) ($P = 0.0008$) at 2nd visit compared to 1st visit. The mean of fractional variation of test-retest to the longitudinal variation was 32%, suggesting data variation does not contribute significantly to the longitudinal observations. Significant correlations were observed in the same parameters measured at both visits including washout time, upslope, overshoot, forward flow time T_{ff}, thoracoabdominal, iliofemoral and total PWVs (all with $r > 0.4$, $P < 0.01$). Correlational analysis among parameters between 1st visit and 2nd visits showed significant influences ($r > 0.29$, $P < 0.05$) of the small venous reactivity parameters (i.e., washout, upslope and overshoot) at 1st visit on the arterial stiffness parameters (aortic arch, thoracoabdominal and iliofemoral PWVs) at follow-ups. Significant correlations between MRI parameters and cardiovascular risk factors were found ($|r| > 0.2$, $P < 0.05$) at longitudinal follow-up visit, as well as between cardiovascular risk factors at 1st visit and MRI parameters at 2nd visit. In conclusion, the vascular reactivity parameters in this study demonstrated significantly worsening of microvascular circulation and arterial stiffness with age and in smokers at 18-month follow-ups. These alterations are more likely to be resulted from atherosclerosis and cardiovascular risk increments over time in especially smokers and elderly people.

Chapter 4 - Prior studies have shown that the hazard ratio increases linearly with the number of risk factors, including cerebrovascular disease, tau and amyloid burden. In this chapter, we will report the longitudinal changes of molecular imaging tracers including tau, amyloid and [^{18}-F]Fluoro-2-deoxyglucose (FDG) quantifications from the ADNI cohort in addition to our previous baseline aging effects findings. Regarding MRI and PET imaging correlations, our aims are to compare the white matter (WM) lesion volume, amyloid burden, FDG glucose uptake in patients with early Alzheimer's disease (AD), mild cognitive impairment (MCI) and healthy controls. And the correlations among WM lesion volume with amyloid burden, FDG uptake as well as functional connectivity changes in MCI and early AD patients will be examined further. Longitudinal tau changes (0.1-1.5% yearly rate of increment) demonstrated a posterior to anterior occipito-temporal degradation pattern at different follow-up times in comparison to baseline. All longitudinal results indicated most significant progression of tau deposition was present in the Braak stage IV regions including temporal pole and middle temporal cortex. Decrement of tau deposition in the early transentorhinal region and fusiform at follow-ups could possibly due to the spreading effects from these earlier Braak stage regions (I & III) to relatively later stage regions such as temporal poles. Significant longitudinal changes of regional amyloid deposition demonstrated about 0.3-0.4% beta-amyloid increment at 24-month follow-up times in the temporal cortex, especially in the middle and inferior temporal sub-segments, compared to baseline. The whole brain cerebrum had about 0.1% increment including regions of bilateral parsorbitalis (about 0.45% biyearly rate) and right lateral occipital cortex (0.15% rate). As for FDG glucose metabolism, longitudinal data found significant reductions (most of $P \leq 0.0001$) of glucose metabolic rate at variable follow-up times in the regions of bilateral temporal, angular and posterior cortices. The rate of FDG metabolism decline varied slightly for different regions, with about -1.6% every year decline of glucose metabolic rate for the posterior cingulum and -1.3% yearly for left temporal cortex, -1.9% yearly for bilateral angular region. Based on ADNI2 cohort data, there is no longitudinal change of global white matter hyperintensity at 3 to 24 months time interval compared to baseline ($P > 0.05$). Regarding the correlations between different imaging parameters, aside from significant associations between tau and other imaging metrics, significant correlation was found between white matter lesion load (WMLL) and amyloid load averaged over the whole cerebral cortex in all three groups combining controls, MCI and AD (Pearson $r = 0.46$, $P = 0.015$; Spearman rank $r = 0.46$, $P = 0.013$). A negative correlation between FDG uptake and amyloid load was noted in all three groups ($r = -0.57$, $P = 0.0006$).

Taken together, there are variable degrees of longitudinal changes regarding to higher tau deposition, amyloid accumulation and FDG hypometabolism with age. The concurrence of WM hyperintensity, gray matter atrophy, structural disconnectivity and functional hyper-perfusion as well as higher tau, amyloid and lower FDG in entorhinal, hippocampal and other temporal regions suggested detectable pathological, structural and functional brain changes at both molecular and macroscopic levels, at even early stages of dementia including MCI patients.

Chapter 5 - Maintaining good metabolic profile plays a significant role in improving the quality of life at aging. Widely recommended physical and psychological strategies include exercise, calorie restriction (such as healthy diet), anti-aging neuroprotective and anti-inflammation therapy. Most occurring risks at middle age range ([45-65] years old) are obesity, insulin resistance, inflammation, alterations in the activity of the hypothalamus-hypophysis suprarenal axis, stress and hypertension that could increase the prevalence of metabolic syndrome. Metabolic syndrome increases with age and particularly for women. Significant associations were seen between imaging measures and cardiovascular risk factors at both baseline and 18-month follow-ups. An example of significant correlations between longitudinal MRI vascular reactivity parameter- hyperemia duration and cardiovascular biomarkers including high-density cholesterol, C-reactive protein, triglycerides and body mass index is given. Physical exercise, healthy diet and calorie restriction therapy as well as arts training could be some promising prevention strategies to reduce and modify the atherosclerosis and cardiovascular risks, as well as help preserve working memory and executive function at aging. Together with accurate imaging evidence, early detection and treatment could be achieved with the ultimate goal of improving quality of life at middle age and extending longevity.

Chapter 1

REVIEW OF MULTI-MODALITIES NEUROIMAGING

ABSTRACT

Longitudinal studies can be used for causality inference based on the temporal orders and correlations among multiple parameters at different time points. Accounting for individual differences including demographic and biological factors is another advantage of longitudinal investigation that uses individual baseline and usually applies paired statistical examination between baseline and follow-ups for the same subject population. Early detection and prevention play a crucial role in treatment and improvement of brain health, and literatures related to longitudinal neuroimaging studies with age are limited. Furthermore, identifying longitudinal changes of neuroimaging parameters at short interval (for instances, 6 months to 72 months) could help determining disease phase (acute vs. chronic), quantifying trajectories of disease progression (early vs. late stage), and prediction of long-term aging-related effects with more complementary health profile. It is important to illustrate the dynamic profiles of blood flow, oxygen utilization (i.e., extraction fraction) as well as glucose, lipid and oxidative metabolism both regionally and globally to better understand the underlying brain functions and physiology with aging. For the past few years, multiple applications of the integrated PET/MRI imaging including inflammation, functional metabolism and microstructure mapping have been reported. The aim of this chapter is to review multi-modality neuroimaging technique and applications, and introduce the main topics of this book-longitudinal imaging and applications in aging and dementia.

It is well known that maintaining brain functional active and metabolic equilibrium is important to a healthy brain and especially for people with age. For instance, cerebral blood flow (CBF) to cerebral metabolic rate of oxygen ($CMRO_2$) coupling decrement and cerebral metabolic rate of glucose (CMRglu) reduction had been observed at normal aging. However, several metabolic and cardiovascular risks increase with age as well, including insulin resistance increment possibly due to hypertension and disrupted glucose/insulin metabolism that are correlated with blood metabolites such as microtubule associated protein (MAP), triglycerides (TG) and high-density cholesterol (HDL) (Craft and Christen, 2009). Thus it is important to illustrate the dynamic profiles of blood flow, oxygen utilization (i.e., extraction fraction) as well as glucose, lipid and oxidative metabolism both regionally and globally to better understand the underlying brain functions and physiology with aging (Lewis and Keshari, 2018). More detailed quantifications of the coupling effects of multiple neurovascular, neurometabolic, oxidative phosphorylation, and vascular-metabolic processes at normal aging and deficits in neurodegenerative disorder including Alzheimer's disease (AD) and diabetes are needed. Improvement of detection of glucose level and insulin signaling pathways using upfront methods at normal aging and under disease conditions such as metabolic syndrome and memory disorders are expected nowadays given the increasing prevalence of these syndromes at early age starting about 40 years old.

Different types of imaging metrics including metabolism, blood velocity and flow rate, oxygen extraction fraction (OEF) and blood-oxygenation-level dependent signal (BOLD) are all inter-connected. For instance, the MRI BOLD effect is well known to result from multiple physiological parametric changes including $CMRO_2$, CBF, OEF and cerebral blood volume (CBV) (Ugurbil et al. 2015). As outlined in the balloon model, the fMRI signals evolve temporally including the initial dip and post-stimulus undershoot, due to different dynamic fractional contributions of CBF, CBV and $CMRO_2$ (Buxton 2002). Utilization of multiple imaging metrics in brain could help us answer the questions of whether and how much the excess CBF change is due to the energy consumption demand ("feedback" model) or is in response to the increased neuronal activity as reflected by $CMRO_2$ change (more towards a "feed-forward" model), and which factors (e.g., brain reserve or vascular reactivity) determine the extent of such changes (Buxton et al. 2012).

Innovative medical imaging equipments such as PET/MRI opens new horizons in multi-parametric and molecular imaging for clinical research that allows simultaneous quantifications of several parameters and underlying pathological mechanisms such as amyloid, tau and glucose metabolism at the same time. While MRI could provide superior structural information, applying MRI anatomical priors to reduce the PET partial volume effect could be achieved to improve spatial resolution of PET images for clinical and research usages. The PET/MRI scanner might help address these issues with advantages of reduced scan time and simultaneous nature of data acquisition. For the past few years, various applications of the integrated PET/MRI imaging including inflammation, functional metabolism and microstructure mapping have been reported (Zhou 2016a; Zhou 2016b). Further applications in brain tumors and cancer response monitoring have reported complementary and valid information that this innovative modality could achieve based on newly developed techniques. Efficient and more accurate imaging technique such as MRI-based attenuation correction (AC) using zero TE (ZTE) for automatic and simplified bone-related tissue signal detection as well as faster and parallel imaging reconstruction has been reported (Larson et al., 2016; Delso et al., 2016; Hitz et al., 2014; Sekine et al., 2016). Advanced MRI-based motion correction for PET image reconstruction, newer PET time of flight reconstruction and incorporation with compressed sensing technique have offered superior temporal and spatial resolutions for disease diagnosis and prevention (Bai et al., 2014; Catana, 2015; Dutta et al., 2015). We had previously briefly reviewed the applications of PET/MRI in neurology with two examples in AD and brain tumor cases (Zhou 2016b).

For instance, numerous imaging studies in AD have been performed to study characteristic brain alterations including brain atrophy with earlier involvement of medial temporal lobe (Rusinek et al., 2004), brain hypo-perfusion in the posterior cingulate and parietal regions (Chao et al., 2010), reduced functional and structural connectivity in the default mode network (DMN) based on MRI findings (Zhou et al., 2008) and hypo-metabolism based on PET imaging findings (Silverman et al., 2004). A regional coupling between metabolism of glucose (via PET kinetic analysis) and CBF had been reported with reductions post-caffeine compared to pre-caffeine conditions in controls (Wang et al., 2011), and in demented patients (Musiek et al., 2012) based on stand-alone scans. An evaluation of the real-time coupling of these two key imaging parameters with simultaneous acquisitions had not been performed before. For example, FDG metabolism had been found to increase twice as the energy brain activation needs (i.e., larger change in metabolism than change in CBF), and at a later time the unmetabolited fraction of the tracer was cleared off so that the tissue concentration of the tracer could reflect the metabolic rate (Buxton 2002; Buxton et al., 1998). Neurovascular coupling between neurochemistry (e.g., dopamine receptor occupancy) and hemodynamic change (e.g., cerebral blood volume) using simultaneous PET/fMRI acquisitions had been reported recently with similar temporal profile and dose response in non-human primates (Sander et al., 2013). Translational studies of neurovascular and neuro-metabolic coupling effects in human beings and patients remain challenging due to inter-subject variability and lack of control template (Zhou et al., 2012b). Despite these challenges, the integrated PET/MRI scanner gained popularity due to some advantages including intrinsic between-modality image registration and better interpretation of underlying co-existing pathophysiological processes (Bai et al., 2013). We had quantified evaluated the most up-to-date PET/MRI scanner performance with multiple functional and structural metrics together with application demonstrations. The integrated PET/MRI images showed comparable image quality to stand-alone imaging modality (both MRI and PET) with the gains of simultaneous multi-parametric acquisitions, reduced scan time and potential patient discomfort. Furthermore, tight correlation between blood flow and metabolism was found in several brain gray matter regions including the temporal lobe in patients (Zhou 2016a).

Tumor growth typically requires new blood vessel formation, causing changes in neurovascular and neurometabolic effects including blood brain barrier (BBB) permeability, blood flow and metabolism (Hutterer et al., 2015). Typical microstructure alteration of tumor characteristics includes changes of diffusion of cell density of tumors and extracellular space narrowing and restricted diffusion properties compared to surrounding tissue types. For instance, using multiple imaging metrics obtained from the integrated PET/MRI scanner, representative images of MRI T1, CBF and PET- FDG uptake of a possible benign tumor case and a glioblastoma multiforme case were illustrated (Zhou 2016b). Compared to benign tumor patient, the glioblastoma patient showed abnormal hyperintensity on T1, hyperperfusion and increased FDG uptake in the affected area. This study described the convenience and feasibility of using simultaneous MRI and PET modality to characterize structural, functional, and molecular signatures of brain tumor. Further study with more subjects and an automatic multi-imaging feature classification to obtain an objective integrated score to predict disease survival rate and recurrence are expected in the future (Hutterer et al., 2015) for the relatively new integrated PET/MRI scanner. Longitudinal monitoring of disease progression at several time points by utilizing subjects' own baseline template and reducing inter-subject variability could overcome some challenges together with the new imaging equipments.

LONGITUDINAL IMAGING AND APPLICATIONS IN AGING AND DEMENTIA

Applications of new imaging probes and correlations with other co-occurring functional and structural imaging findings together with biological data of aging brain and memory disorder are of importance to improve early dementia detection as well as to maintain optimal memory function. Recent accumulating evidence indicates that each neuroimaging modality can provide unique imaging features; and multi-parametric imaging methods could help better interpret functional/structural changes in memory and dementia. Together with the phenotypic and genetic data, these multi-parametric diagnosis metrics could innovate the early dementia field of staging and prevention. With the advanced functional, structural and molecular imaging techniques, we can identify subtle neuroplastic and neuropathological changes in early Alzheimer's disease (AD) that are not seen using traditional methods and could correlate better with the underlying pathological mechanism. Adjustment for these confounding factors including clinical and genetic data and acquisition of longitudinal data to elucidate the causality effects and better staging of memory disorder at early stage and even for participants at middle age with different imaging biomarkers are the potential strategies.

Investigating brain changes with each neuroimaging metric at aging and their rates of changes at relatively short interval are of importance since many age-related risks such as cardiovascular burden and neuroinflammation increases at age and could confound baseline results (Thakur and Rattan, 2012). Longitudinal studies can be used for causality inference based on the temporal orders and correlations among multiple parameters at different time points. Accounting for individual differences including demographic and biological factors is another advantage of longitudinal investigation that uses individual baseline and usually applies paired statistical examination between baseline and follow-ups for the same subject population. Early detection and prevention play a crucial role in treatment and improvement of brain health; however, literatures related to longitudinal neuroimaging studies with age are limited. Furthermore, identifying longitudinal changes of neuroimaging parameters at short interval (for instances, 6 months to 72 months) could help determining the disease phase (acute vs. chronic), quantifying trajectories of disease progression (early vs. late stage), and prediction of long-term aging-related effects with more complementary health profile (Weiner et al., 2017). Finally, longitudinal monitoring and advanced analyses of complete multi-parametric imaging quantifications in large cohort subject population is one of the topics of big data and remains as the focus of clinical research that could expand our horizons to the next era of personal and precise medicine.

In this book, longitudinal neuroimaging changes of structural and functional connectivities using both diffusion tensor imaging and functional connectivity with MRI (fcMRI) techniques will be examined thoroughly. Longitudinal changes of neurocognitive function tests and their correlations with neuroimaging metrics will be investigated further. Effects of age and smoking on the endothelial function measured with MRI vascular reactivity will be demonstrated at both baseline and longitudinal follow-ups. Intra- and inter- correlations among multiple MRI parameters and with cardiovascular factors at each visit as well as between two visits will be performed to illustrate the causality and influence of each parameter. Longitudinal changes of PET molecular imaging parameters for neuropathological quantification including amyloid accumulation, tau deposition and glucose metabolism will be quantified based on data from Alzheimer's disease neuroimaging initiative (ADNI) cohort in addition to the baseline findings of aging effects and differentiation of multiple preclinical and early dementia stages. Correlations between MRI metrics such as white matter hyperintensity and functional activity with several pathological burdens measured with PET will be evaluated further. Some promising prevention strategies of metabolism syndrome such as physical exercise, healthy diet and calorie restriction therapy as well as arts training to modify and reduce the atherosclerosis and cardiovascular risks will be reviewed. And finally, early detection of dementia and metabolic syndrome with advanced imaging techniques for prevention at early middle age and delaying disease onset will be proposed and investigated.

REFERENCES

[1] Bai B, Li Q, Leahy RM. Magnetic resonance-guided positron emission tomography image reconstruction. *Seminars in nuclear medicine*. 2013; 43(1): 30-44.

[2] Bai, B, et al. MAP reconstruction for Fourier rebinned TOF-PET data. *Phys Med Biol*. 2014; 59, 925-949, doi:10.1088/0031-9155/59/4/925.

[3] Burris, NS et al. Detection of Small Pulmonary Nodules with Ultrashort Echo Time Sequences in Oncology Patients by Using a PET/MR System. *Radiology*. 2016; 278: 239-246.

[4] Buxton RB. Dynamic models of BOLD contrast. *NeuroimageI* 2012; 62(2): 953-961.

[5] Buxton RB. *Introduction to Functional Magnetic Resonance Imaging - Principles & Techniques.* Cambridge University Press. 2002.

[6] Buxton RB, Frank LR, Wong EC, Siewert B, Warach S, Edelman RR. A general kinetic model for quantitative perfusion imaging with arterial spin labeling. *Magnetic resonance in medicine*:

official journal of the Society of Magnetic Resonance in Medicine/Society of Magnetic Resonance in Medicine. 1998; 40(3): 383-396.

[7] Catana, C. Motion correction options in PET/MRI. *Semin Nucl Med.* 2015; 45: 212-223.

[8] Chao LL, Buckley ST, Kornak J, et al. ASL perfusion MRI predicts cognitive decline and conversion from MCI to dementia. *Alzheimer disease and associated disorders*. 2010; 24(1):19-27.

[9] Craft S and Christen Y. *Diabetes, Insulin and Alzheimer's Disease*. Springer. 2009.

[10] Delso, G, et al. Effect of Time-of-Flight Information on PET/MR Reconstruction Artifacts: Comparison of Free-breathing versus Breath-hold MR-based Attenuation Correction. *Radiology,* 152509, doi:10.1148/radiol.2016152509 (2016).

[11] Dutta, J., Huang, C., Li, Q. & El Fakhri, G. Pulmonary imaging using respiratory motion compensated simultaneous PET/MR. *Med Phys* 42, 4227-4240, doi:10.1118/1.4921616 (2015).

[12] Frietsch T, Maurer MH, Vogel J, Gassmann M, Kuschinsky W, Waschke KF. Reduced cerebral blood flow but elevated cerebral glucose metabolic rate in erythropoietin overexpressing transgenic mice with excessive erythrocytosis. *Journal of cerebral blood flow and metabolism: official journal of the International Society of Cerebral Blood Flow and Metabolism* 2007;27(3):469-476.

[13] Fox PT, Raichle ME, Mintun MA, Dence C. Nonoxidative glucose consumption during focal physiologic neural activity. *Science* 1988; 241(4864): 462-464.

[14] Hall, H, et al. Distribution of D1- and D2-dopamine receptors, and dopamine and its metabolites in the human brain. *Neuropsychopharmacology.* 1994;11:245-256.

[15] Hitz, S, et al. Systematic Comparison of the Performance of Integrated Whole-Body PET/MR Imaging to Conventional PET/CT for (1)(8)F- FDG Brain Imaging in Patients Examined for Suspected Dementia. *J Nucl Med.* 2014; 55: 923-931.

[16] Hutterer et al. Current standards and new concepts in MRI and PET response assessment of antiangiogenic therapies in high-grade glioma patients. *Neuro Oncology.* 2015; 17(6):784.

[17] Kamil Ugurbil, Lawrence Berliner, Kamil Uludag, *FMRI: From Nuclear Spins to Brain Functions,* Springer, 2015.

[18] Larson, PE, et al. Ultrashort echo time and zero echo time MRI at 7T. *MAGMA.* 2016; 29(3): 359-370.

[19] Laruelle, M, et al. SPECT quantification of [123I]iomazenil binding to benzodiazepine receptors in nonhuman primates: I. Kinetic modeling of single bolus experiments. *J Cereb Blood Flow Metab.* 1994; 14:439-452, doi:10.1038/jcbfm.1994.55.

[20] Lewis JS and Keshari KR, *Imaging and Metabolism*, Springer, 2018.

[21] Musiek ES, Chen Y, Korczykowski M, et al. Direct comparison of fluorodeoxyglucose positron emission tomography and arterial spin labeling magnetic resonance imaging in Alzheimer's disease. *Alzheimer's & dementia: The journal of the Alzheimer's Association.* 2012; 8(1): 51-59.

[22] Rusinek H, Endo Y, De Santi S, et al. Atrophy rate in medial temporal lobe during progression of Alzheimer disease. *Neurology.* 2004; 63(12): 2354-2359.

[23] Sander CY, Hooker JM, Catana C, et al. *Neurovascular coupling to D2/D3 dopamine receptor occupancy using simultaneous PET/ functional MRI.* Proc Natl Acad Sci U S A. 2013.

[24] Sekine T, Ter Voert EE, Warnock G, et al. Clinical evaluation of ZTE attenuation correction for brain FDG-PET/MR imaging-comparison with atlas attenuation correction. *J Nucl Med.* 2016; June.

[25] Silverman DH, Small GW, Phelps ME. Clinical Value of Neuroimaging in the Diagnosis of Dementia. Sensitivity and Specificity of Regional Cerebral Metabolic and Other Parameters for Early Identification of Alzheimer's Disease. *Clinical positron*

imaging: official journal of the Institute for Clinical PET. 1999; 2(3):119-130.

[26] Wang DJ, Chen Y, Fernandez-Seara MA, Detre JA. Potentials and challenges for arterial spin labeling in pharmacological magnetic resonance imaging. *The Journal of pharmacology and experimental therapeutics*. 2011; 337(2):359-366.

[27] Weiner MW, Veitch DP, Aisen PS, et al., Recent publications from the Alzheimer's Disease Neuroimaging Initiative: Reviewing progress toward improved AD clinical trials, *Alzheimer's & Dementia*. 2017; 13:e1-e85.

[28] Zhou Y, Dougherty JH, Jr., Hubner KF, Bai B, Cannon RL, Hutson RK. Abnormal connectivity in the posterior cingulate and hippocampus in early Alzheimer's disease and mild cognitive impairment. *Alzheimer's & dementia: The journal of the Alzheimer's Association* 2008;4(4):265-270.

[29] Zhou Y, Quantitative mMR (PET/MRI) Evaluation and Application in Dementia, *Jacobs Journal of Medical Diagnosis and Medical Imaging*, Editorial. 2016a; 1(1).

[30] Zhou Y, *Functional Neuroimaging with Multiple Modalities: Principles, Device and Applications,* Nova Science Publishers. 2016b.

Chapter 2

LONGITUDINAL CHANGES OF STRUCTURAL AND FUNCTIONAL CONNECTIVITY AT AGING AND CORRELATIONS WITH GENETICS AND NEUROCOGNITIVE METRICS

ABSTRACT

Revealing brain functional and micro-structural changes over a relatively short period at individual levels are especially important given that many risks associated with age including vascular-metabolism and neuroinflammation increases and could confound the baseline fMRI parametric images. Cellular-level axonal injury and/or demyelination as well as dispersed mesoscopic level substance abnormal aggregation and structural/functional abnormality could occur in short subacute/acute phases. Literatures related to longitudinal changes with age are limited while only a few studies reported. In addition to our previous fMRI findings, longitudinal data including diffusion tensor imaging (DTI) and functional activity were used to characterize multiple neuroimaging parameters including random intercept and interval per individual together with genetic data and neurocognitive tests. The correlations among different imaging metrics as well as between neuroimaging findings and neurocognitive scores were further quantified. No significant age by gender interactions have been found to either DTI fractional anisotropy (FA) or diffusivity metrics. The interval effective regions showed longitudinal change of FA and radial diffusivity (RD)/axial diffusivity (AX) values remained similar to the aging results found with baseline data. Significant correlations between DTI and fMRI metrics as well as between imaging and neurocognitive data including speed and memory were found. Our results indicate significant and consistent age, gender and apolipoprotein E (APOE) genotypic effects on structural and functional connectivities at both short interval and baseline, in addition to correlational neurocognitive functions.

Keywords: microstructure, function connectivity, DTI, longitudinal change, neurocognitive test, correlation, age, APOE gene

1. Introduction

Functional connectivity based on MRI (fcMRI) measures simultaneous and synchronous neuronal activities at various regions connected intrinsically in brain with functional MRI time courses. In our recent study, we reported lower functional connectivity in posterior cingulate and temporal regions with aging within the default mode network (DMN) (Zhou 2016). We also found higher fcMRI in the dorso-attentional network (DAN) at aging, which could be due to the negative connectivity with DMN. Furthermore longitudinal changes in fcMRI occurred in regions similar to those demonstrating cross-sectional effects of age with less significance level, and only a few small brain areas showing significant age by interval or gender by interval effects. The rate of fcMRI longitudinal change, however, was not influenced significantly by baseline age or gender, after adjusting for baseline age and gender modulation effects in majority of brain regions, suggesting moderate linear interval effects of fcMRI longitudinal changes in brain. Our results form this relatively large cohort suggest that fcMRI variability from various networks in different scales might be useful to monitor brain changes in normal aging and preclinical stages of Alzheimer's disease (Zhou 2016). As for diffusion tensor imaging (DTI), both voxel-wise four DTI metrics and tract-specific ROI analysis were used to investigate myelin and axonal integrity differences with age, gender and APOE genotype at baseline (Huster et al. 2002; Basser 1995; Zhou 2004; Thiessen et al. 2013). One of our main findings was the decreased fractional anisotropy (FA) but increased radial diffusivity (RD) with age based on both voxel-wise and tract-specific analyses (Zhou 2016), indicating both axonal degeneration and demyelination (Billiet et al. 2015; Bazes et al. 2016). Dramatic decreases of FA with age, especially in participants over 50 years old, accompanied by increased RD suggest that white matter (WM) integrity declines with age. In contrast, changes in axial diffusivity (AX) and mean diffusivity (MD) with age are in two-way: higher AX and MD in some tracts and cortical regions including bilateral thalamic radiation and cingulum bundles, as well as decreased AX and MD in some long-distance fasciculus (Sasson et al. 2012; Agosta et al. 2014; Kochunov et al. 2011; Horch et al. 2011).

Regarding DTI and fMRI correlations, significant gray matter (GM) and WM correspondences based on GM atrophy and WM fractional anisotropy (FA) reductions in several brain regions were found in multiple sclerosis (MS) patients including primary visual cortex/optic radiation as well as somatosensory cortex/superior longitudinal fasciculus at baseline (Zhou 2017b). However, with disease progresses, these associations might be deteriorated and are not maintained although each imaging feature remains consistent and highly correlated at multiple baseline and longitudinal time points (Kolasa et al. 2015; Rocca et al. 2016). The degree of change (or rate of change) of each metric is dependent on the sensitivity during the disease course (Forn et al. 2007; Lowe et al. 2008; Lisak et al. 2007). For instance, GM atrophy and functional coordination decrement were found at follow-up visit in MS patients, in contrast to the baseline observation of significant FA reductions and WM lesions predominantly in corpus callosum, periventricular areas, occipital horns and cingulum areas at baseline in MS compared to controls (Zhou 2017b). In mild traumatic brain injury (MTBI), one year after injury, there was measurable global brain atrophy, with a degree larger than control subjects. The anterior cingulate WM bilaterally and the left cingulate gyrus isthmus WM, as well as the right precuneal GM, showed significant decreases in regional volume in patients with MTBI over the 1st year after injury (Yount et al. 2002). However at baseline, after normalization to supratentorial brain volume, there were no significant regional brain volume differences between patients with MTBI at the time of their initial visit and the control group. Our observations complement these findings and indicate that specific brain structure such as the cingulum and precuneus may be more vulnerable to long-term structural changes (Hudak et al. 2011; Zhou 2017a).

It had been reported that baseline imaging findings including micro-structure integrity measured with DTI can predict functional activation and coordination at follow-ups (Bendfeldt et al. 2009; Bjartmar et al. 2003; Bodini et al. 2009). We had reported that FA measure at baseline predicted follow-up functional coordination score from fMRI data ($r = 0.68$, $P = 0.007$), indicating a possible initial WM inflammatory factor to the subsequent neurodegenerative processes in MS patients (Zhou 2017b). We also found that baseline composite imaging metrics can predict follow-up cognitive function and neuropsychological scores (Zhou 2017a). For instance, in MTBI, the clinical symptom at 1-year follow-up visit could be predicted with high accuracy from baseline imaging features with $r = -0.82$, $P < 0.001$ for depression; $r = -0.65$, $P = 0.01$ for anxiety; $r = -0.71$, $P = 0.005$ for fatigue; and $r = -0.67$, $P = 0.008$ for post-concussion syndrome (PCS) (Zhou 2017a). Revealing the brain micro-structural changes over a relatively short period at individual levels are especially important given that many risks associated with age including vascular and neuroinflammation increases and could confound the baseline parametric images of each individual. However, literatures related to longitudinal changes of neuroimaging data with age are limited with only a few reported findings (Bender and Raz 2015).

The goals of this study are to assess baseline and longitudinal age, gender-related as well as apolipoprotein E (APOE) genotypic effects with neuroimaging and neurocognitive data from a large sample of healthy older adults. The strengths of this study are the extensive and well-characterized large sample of older adults, and multiple imaging metrics including advanced fcMRI, four DTI (FA, MD, RD, AX) metrics to capture extensive properties of functional connectivity and white matter myelination at both baseline and longitudinal follow-up time points. Both conventional whole brain voxel-wise analyses and fiber track-specific ROI quantification measures that are more robust and less prone to registration error were used to increase the white matter myelin detection specificity. In addition to previous fcMRI findings (Zhou 2016), we also investigate longitudinal changes of multiple DTI and fMRI metrics using advanced linear mixed effects (LME) statistical model, together with neurocognitive tests. The correlations among different imaging metrics as well as between neuroimaging findings and neurocognitive scores were quantified to better illustrate the full spectrum of multiple phenotypic data.

2. METHODS

2.1. Participants

We studied 572 cognitively normal participants in the neuroimaging substudy from the Baltimore Longitudinal Study of Aging (BLSA) who had DTI assessments. Exclusion criteria were as follows: subjects with excessive motions and unwanted imaging qualities (N = 17 and 30 scans); subjects with incidental findings of brain lesions or other central nervous diseases such as Parkinson's disease (N = 4). 21 individuals aged 24-39, 39 individuals aged 40-49, 51 aged 50-59, 137 aged 60-69, 186 aged 70-79, and 138 aged 80-89.

387 participants (68%) had available APOE genotype information, 107 APOE ε4+ and 280 APOE ε4- participants were further divided into 6 sub-groups based on the APOE isoforms. These sample characteristics are shown in Table 1. 245 subjects had longitudinal DTI follow-up (interval range 0.9-3.5 years, mean interval of 1.9 ± 0.6 years) and were used to characterize aging effects at short interval. fcMRI studies with 608 baseline and 278 longitudinal follow-up participants were described in our recent work (Zhou 2016). 236 participants had both fMRI and DTI scans and were used for correlation analysis (Table 1, rightmost column). Neurocognitive data from 21 cognitive tests with 59 variables that measure multiple cognitive functionalities, including visual perception and attention, learning ability, memory encoding and recall, language fluency, and executive function, for each participant were collected at the same day of the MRI scan (McCarrey et al. 2016). After post-processing with statistical normalization database, 52 test Z-scores were used for further analysis including longitudinal LME and correlational analysis.

Table 1. Participants characteristics at baseline and six APOE genotypic sub-groups including both DTI and fMRI scans

Characteristic	All DTI Baseline	ε4/ε4	ε3/ε4	ε2/ε4	ε3/ε3	ε2/ε3	ε2/ε2	Both DTI and fMRI
Total n	572	4	95	8	219	59	2	236
age, years; mean ± SD	69.7 ± 13.4	68.4 ± 16.8	67.0 ± 12.1	69.4 ± 12.6	70.1 ± 11.3	70.0 ± 10.1	75.9 ± 16.4	72.0 ± 12.2
Gender n; women/men	311/261	3/1	56/39	7/1	115/104	30/29	1/1	135/101
Education, years; mean ± SD	17.1 ± 2.7	17.5 ± 1.0	17.4 ± 2.5	17.1 ± 2.1	16.9 ± 2.6	17.6 ± 2.2	16.0 ± 2.8	17.0 ± 2.4
MMSE at visit	28.6 ± 1.5	28.3 ± 1.5	28.8 ± 1.4	29.5 ± 0.6	28.4 ± 1.6	28.5 ± 1.4	29.0 ± 1.4	28.8 ± 1.3

2.2. Imaging Parameters

MRI imaging was obtained with a 3T whole-body scanner (Philips, Achieva) at National Institute of Aging, using an 8-channel head coil. The DTI sequence was evaluated previously and found to have good intra-site reliability and inter-section reproducibility (Zhou 2016). Specifically, standard echo-planar imaging (EPI)-based DTI protocol was performed during the routine 45-minutes scan (TR/TE = 6801/75 msec, flip angle = 90°, FOV = 212x212mm^2, spatial resolution = 0.83x0.83x2.2 mm^3, 65 slices to cover the whole cerebrum). 32 diffusion gradient directions (diffusion gradient time Δ = 36.3ms and pulse duration δ = 16ms) with b-factor of 700 s/mm^2 and a total of 3:58 min for each run as well as two identical runs were obtained for each subject.

A standard EPI resting-state (RS)-fMRI protocol (TR/TE = 2000/30 msec, flip angle = 75°, FOV = 240x240 mm^2, voxel size = 3x3x4 mm^3, 37 slices) was performed during an approximately 45-minute brain MRI protocol. A total of 180 volumes were acquired during the 6-min RS-fMRI scan. Participants were instructed to remain still, with eyes open and focused on a cross fixation, and encouraged to relax during the scan. A 3-dimensional T1-weighted MPRAGE (magnetization prepared rapid gradient-echo imaging) sequence (TR/TE/TI = 6.8/3.2/849.2 msec, FA = 8°, FOV = 192x256x256 mm^3, voxel size = 1.2x1x1 mm^3) was acquired in sagittal-view for segmentation of tissue types and registration/ normalization of EPI images to MNI space.

2.3. Image Processing

DTI data were first pre-processed with the Diffusion Toolkit toolbox (http://trackvis.org) to obtain the four metrics-FA/RD/AX/MD values in original b0 space. For the FA/RA/AD/MD quantification, the

FMRIB, Software Library (FSL, http://fsl.fmrib.ox.ac.uk/fsl) tract-based spatial statistics toolbox steps 1–2 (i.e., preprocessing, brain mask extraction with FA > 0.2 and normalization) were used for registration of all participants' FA into the FSL 1-mm white matter skeleton template. The transformation of the individual FA data to the FSL Montreal Neurological Institute (MNI) template with 1-mm isotropic voxel size, was implemented with the nonlinear registration tool FNIRT based on a b-spline representation of the registration warp field. After normalization of FA map to the MNI space, tract-specific mean FA values were obtained in 20 regions from the well-defined probabilistic tract template (FSL/JHU ICBM atlas). Quantitative MD/AX/RD values were obtained by applying the same transformation from individual FA to template space and computed with tract-specific values (Zhou 2016).

The anatomic T1-MPRAGE and 4D EPI functional data were preprocessed using both FSL and Analysis of Functional NeuroImages (AFNI) programs (adapted scripts from http://www.nitrc.org/projects/fcon_1000 developed based on FSL and AFNI). For structural MPRAGE data used for fMRI data normalization, preprocessing included reorientation to the right-posterior-inferior convention and skull stripping, and segmentation into three tissue types: GM, WM, and cerebrospinal fluid (CSF). The segmental tissue masks were used to derive the nuisance fMRI signals in WM and CSF. Finally, the MPRAGE image was co-registered with the fMRI data and normalized to the Montreal Neurological Institute (MNI) 152-brain template with 2-mm isotropic voxel size (Zhou 2016; Zhou 2017b).

For fcMRI processing, the first four volumes of the RS-fMRI data of each subject were discarded for scanner and image stability. Preprocessing steps for RS-fMRI data included rigid alignment of the time frames using AFNI motion correction algorithms, spatial smoothing using a Gaussian kernel with 6 mm full-width- at-half-maximum (FWHM), and band-pass temporal filtering of 0.005–0.1 Hz to improve signal-to-noise ratio. Removal of nuisance signals was then performed using a Gaussian regression model after co-registration to

MPRAGE data. Namely, motion parameters, global signal, and signals derived from CSF and WM based on the tissue masks were modeled in the Gaussian linear mixed model, and residual signal at each voxel was maintained for further analyses. And the residual 4D fMRI data after regression were transformed to MNI standard space (Zhou et al. 2012). A DMN seed including both medial prefrontal cortex (MED) (MNI center: 0, 48, 23 mm) and posterior cingulate cortex (PCC) (MNI center: 26, 248, 39 mm) with a combined volume of 4112 mm^3 (each seed of 2056 mm^3) was used. We refer to this seed as the combined core seed. We chose the combined core seed over separate PCC and MED seeds because the latter approach generates different and incomplete DMN connectivity patterns (Andrews-Hanna et al. 2010), whereas the combined core seed yields consistent and complete depictions of DMN. Whole brain voxel-wise Pearson correlation coefficients were computed between the average time series within the seed and the time course of each fMRI voxel in the brain. Finally Z-statistics were derived voxel-wise. 2nd-level Gaussian random field (GRF) and family-wise corrections were applied to derive the functional connectivity (FC) map with FSL toolbox.

In addition to the combined core seed, the fcMRI generated from other seeds were also evaluated to study the systematic-level fcMRI, with a total of 26 seeds. The other 25 seeds included 12 conventional regions of different sub-areas of DMN (e.g., PCC and intra-parietal sulcus), 3 thalamic (left, right, and whole thalamus) and 7 subthalamic seeds (Zhou et al. 2014), as well as 3 subcortical seeds (caudate and putamen from the MNI template, and hypothalamus from an in-house developed probability map) (Zhou 2017a). The conventional 12 seeds were derived from the script seed library (http://www.nitrc.org /projects/fcon_1000), including the hippocampal formation and frontal eye field (FEF) seeds that generated the task-positive networks (i.e., these networks are more active at task-conditions, in contrast to resting state). All seeds were evaluated and validated previously (Fox and Raichle 2007). The global mean z-values were obtained from the fcMRI maps generated from each of 26 seeds to study age and gender effects as well, by averaging the fcMRI Z-maps over the whole brain with a threshold of GRF cluster-corrected $P < 0.01$.

Meanwhile in the resting state, fractional amplitude of low-frequency fluctuations (fALFF) has been shown to be higher in the DMN regions that are active and it had also been reported that task-related (e.g., working memory, motor visual stimuli and cognitive tasks) alterations of low-frequency oscillations could reflect real-time neuronal activity (Zhou et al. 2014). The idea of fALFF method was to compute the fraction of the amplitude at low-frequency band (e.g., 0.01-0.08Hz) to the summary of amplitude across whole band for the purpose of removing flat white and peak physiological noise. In this study, the resting-state fALFF Z-value at baseline and longitudinal changes of fALFF, as well as correlations with the age and other fcMRI/DTI neuroimaging metrics were performed from 236 participants with available data resource.

2.4. Statistical Analyses

For DTI, effects of age, gender and APOE genotype were studied at both whole-brain voxel-wise level and tract-specific ROI analyses using the four DTI metrics-FA, RD, AX and MD. LME model was applied to characterize both baseline and longitudinal effects of age, gender and age by gender interactions of the four metrics (Zhou 2016; Goh et al. 2012). We used the MATLAB Statistics toolbox (www.mathworks.com, R2015b) and in-house programs to perform model fitting as listed in equation (1). Longitudinal data were incorporated to characterize the longitudinal change of DTI metrics with interval as the prediction parameter as well. In order to account for within-individual correlations stemming from follow-up data, we included random intercept and random interval (i.e., random slope) terms per individual in LME.

$$DTI \sim \beta_0 + \beta_1 \text{gender} + \beta_2 \text{baseage} + \beta_3 \text{interval} + \beta_4 \text{interval} : \text{baseage} + \beta_5 \text{gender} : \text{baseage} + \beta_6 \text{interval} : \text{gender} \quad (1)$$

For whole-brain analyses, voxel-wise linear regression with DTI metrics as the dependent variable and age as an independent variable using SPM12 software (Statistical Parametric Mapping, http://fil.ion.ucl.ac.uk/spm/software/spm12) was implemented. Gender term was included as a covariate. Then two-sample t-test comparison using baseline DTI data was also implemented to study gender differences between women and men, and age was used as a covariate (Zhou 2018).

For tract-specific ROI-based analyses, the mean value of each regional FA and diffusivity (i.e., RD, AX and MD) analysis were quantified with FSL toolbox and in-house programs developed with MATLAB (www.mathematics.com). Both linear and quadratic fitting were used to examine white matter myelination along aging trajectories. Mean values of all six APOE genotypes were derived from each ROI to form the waveform and multiple-group comparisons of the four DTI metrics stratified by genotypic isoforms were performed in MATLAB toolbox.

To characterize baseline and longitudinal changes in fcMRI, we used a LME model, similar to DTI longitudinal data model with the same analyses algorithm as listed in equation (2). In order to account for cross-sectional differences across individuals, we included baseline age (as variable of baseage) and gender as covariates (Zhou 2016). Baseline age was centered at group mean of 69.4 years. Men were coded as 0.5 and women as -0.5. Time interval in years between baseline and follow-up was included to capture longitudinal change in fcMRI. Interaction terms were included with interval, random intercept and interval terms to compute longitudinal rates of fcMRI change accounting for baseline age and gender interactions.

$$fcMRI \sim \beta 0 + \beta 1\ baseage + \beta 2\ gender + \beta 3\ interval + \beta 4\ interval : baseage + \beta 5\ gender : baseage + \beta 6\ interval : gender \quad (2)$$

Conventional statistical comparison (with relatively smaller number of participants) using a two-sample t-test at baseline and two-year follow-ups, adjusting for gender, with the same statistical threshold as in LME model ($P < 0.01$ and cluster size ≥ 10 voxels) was performed for baseline and longitudinal fALFF data quantification. To validate the age and gender effects observed in LME model, SPM-based regression model including general linear correlational analysis between age and fMRI data adjusted for gender, and comparison between women and men group adjusted for age were performed as well.

3. RESULTS

3.1. Age Effects on DTI

Whole brain DTI FA showed prominent aging effects (i.e., reduced FA with aging) in the main projections fibers including cingulum bundle and superior longitudinal fasciculus ($P < 0.00001$) (Figure 1a). The monotonically reduction of FA was observed in relatively older subject with age larger than 50 years old that construe the majority of the sample size. RD, on the other hand, showed only significantly higher RD values with age in bilateral thalamic radiations, bilateral somatosensory cortex, visual cortex, anterior and posterior cingulate gyri, middle temporal cortex including hippocampus, subcallosal cortex and posterior cerebellum ($P < 0.01$, cluster size = 10) (Zhou 2016). Very small clusters and primarily in the cerebellum was found to have lower RD along the age (Figure 1b). Axial diffusivity showed significantly higher values with age in some similar regions to RD including bilateral thalamic radiations, bilateral somatosensory cortex, visual cortex, posterior cerebellum and superior corona radiata tracts ($P < 0.01$, cluster size = 10). In contrast to RD and FA, AX was also significantly lower in white matter regions including bilateral cortico-spinal tract, inferior longitudinal fasciculus, optic radiation and cerebellum (Figure 1c). MD shows almost a similar aging pattern as of AX (Figure 1d) (Zhou 2016).

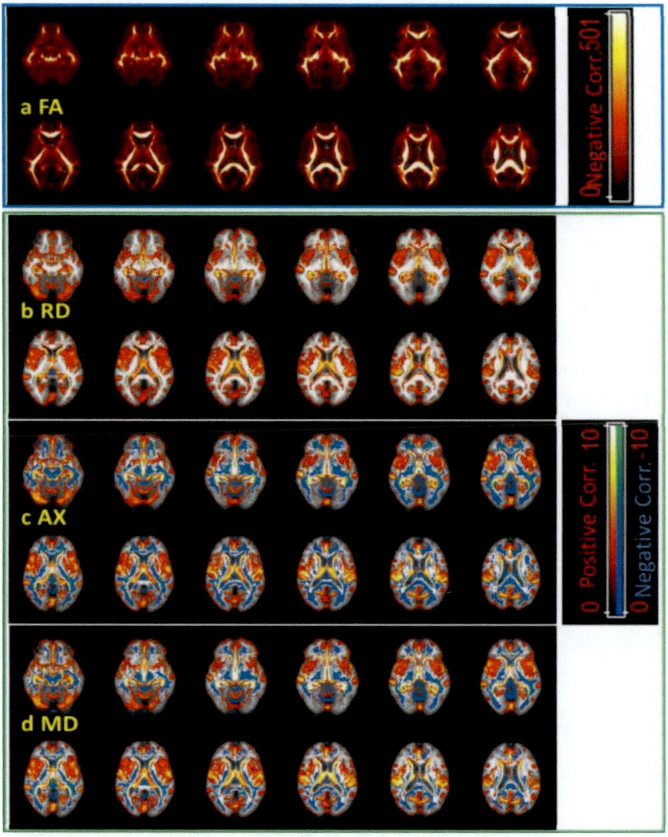

Figure 1. a. Prominent aging effects were demonstrated with negative correlation between voxel-wise FA and age, i.e., decreased FA along the age (statistical T map, $P < 0.01$, cluster size = 10) for all brain regions. On the other hand, RD was increased along the age for some of the brain regions including somatosensory cortex and cingulum bundle (b). There are both increases and decreases of AX (c) and MD (d) along the age, and the changes of AX and MD have very similar patterns (all $P < 0.01$, cluster size = 10). Background image was derived from average of all subjects' FA maps in MNI space.

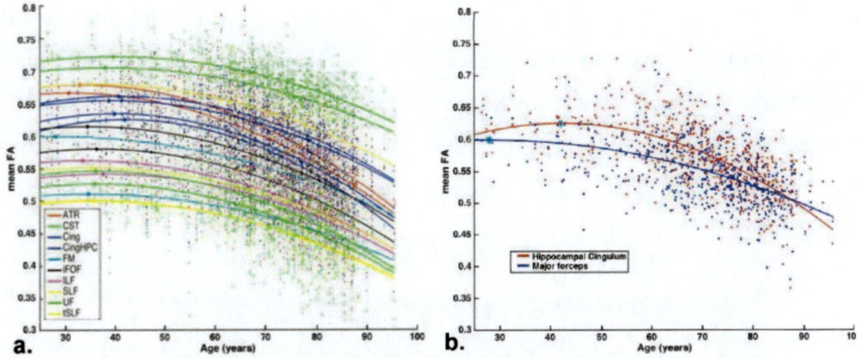

ATR = anterior thalamic radiation; CST = cortico-spinal tract; Cing = cingulum; CingHPC = hippocampal portion of the cingulum bundle; FM = Forceps major and Forceps minor; iFOF = inferior fronto-occipital fasciculus; ILF = inferior longitudinal fasciculus; SLF = superior longitudinal fasciculus; UF = uncinate fasciculus; tSLF = temporal part of superior longitudinal fasciculus. Each color represents bilateral tract-specific FA average on the left and right tracts, except for FM that derives from the average of the forceps major and forceps minor.

Figure 2. a: Quadratic aging trajectories of all 10 tracks with each representing the average FA of left and right tracks, and star (*) indicates maturation age where mean FA of each tract-specific ROI reaches maximum. **b**: Quadratic aging trajectories of two representative tract-specific ROIs. Star (cyan color) indicates maturation age when mean FA of the tract each tract-specific ROI reaches maximum. Major forceps has the earliest maturation age, with highest FA at 27.9 years (blue color). While the left hippocampal portion of the cingulum bundle has the latest maturation age, with highest FA at 42.1 years (red color).

As expected, all the tract-based ROI showed significant aging effects (i.e., reduced FA with age) after adjustment for multiple comparisons ($|r|$ = 0.3-0.7, mean $|r|$ = 0.5, corrected $P < 0.0001$). Quadratic fitting of FA from 20 track-specific ROIs showed aging trajectories with maturation age (i.e., mean FA reaches maximum) falling between [28-42] years. The relatively earlier maturation age was found in the major forceps and bilateral thalamic radiation (28-33 years) and later maturation age from bilateral hippocampal portion of the cingulum and cortico-spinal tracts (39-42 years) (Figure 2a). The tract-based ROI that has the earliest maturation age with highest FA at 27.9 years is the major forceps. The left hippocampal portion of the cingulum bundle has the latest maturation age (42.1 years) (Figure 2b).

While the diffusivity measures from tract-based ROIs showed mostly linearly increases of diffusivity along the age with RD, and some tracts showed no significant aging effects based on AX or MD.

Using Diffusion Toolkit (http://www.nitre.org/projects/trackvis/) with an advanced tensorline propagation algorithm for fiber tracking, we found tracts that play important roles in memory and cognitive function also illustrated significant aging effects. For instance, both fiber tract numbers of the fornix that connects the hippocampus to the whole brain, and fibro bundles connecting bilateral parahippocampus to the whole brain were decreased significantly with aging (both $P < 0.00001$).

3.2. Longitudinal Change of FA

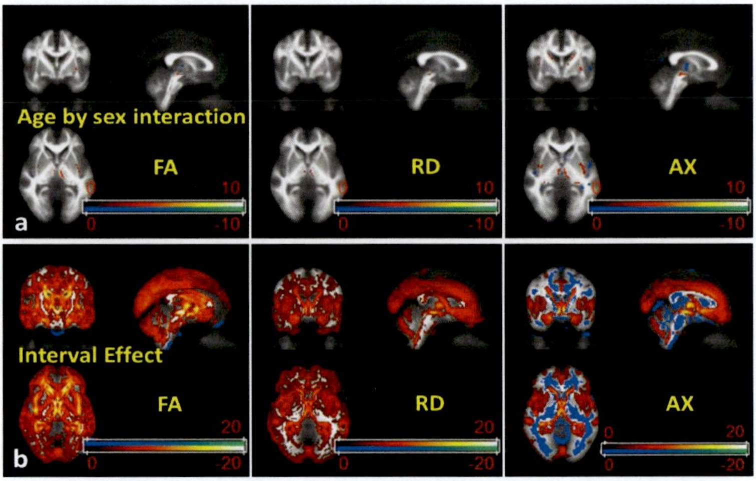

Figure 3. a. Based on LME model, no significant age by gender interaction of DTI FA and diffusivity values across whole-brain with only a few outliers ($P < 0.01$). b. The interval effect estimated from LME model using longitudinal data showed longitudinal change of FA, RD and AX values (MD is almost the same as AX) in brain regions similar to the baseline aging effects (1-3 years of interval of follow-up time; $P < 0.01$, cluster size = 10) with slightly less significance levels, suggesting an observable longitudinal change within a short time interval.

Based on LME model, no significant age by gender interactions have been found to either FA or diffusivity metrics in the whole-brain voxel-wise analyses indicating aging and gender effects can be studied independently (Figure 3a). The interval effective regions estimated from LME model showed longitudinal change of FA, RD and AX values were similar to the aging effect results found with baseline data as in Figure 1 , with slightly less significance levels ($P < 0.01$, cluster size = 10) (Figure 3b).

3.3. Gender Effects on DTI

We found men had significantly higher FA in the hippocampal portion of the cingulum bundle, secondary somatosensory cortex, thalamus, cingulate and cerebellar regions compared to women, based on voxel-wise FA comparisons ($P < 0.01$). Lower FA in men than women in bilateral inferior longitudinal fasciculus, anterior thalamic radiation, frontal cortex and temporal part of the superior longitudinal fasciculus were also observed ($P < 0.01$, cluster size = 10). Higher RD were found in scattered cortical regions including superior frontal, cerebellum and insular in men than women, but lower RD in cerebellar small clusters. Furthermore, AX and MD values were higher in most of brain regions in men than women ($P < 0.01$, cluster size = 10).

3.4. APOE Genotype Effects on DTI and fcMRI

Voxel-wise DTI FA and MD comparisons between different APOE genotypes showed differences in scattered brain clusters ($P < 0.01$, cluster size = 10). Scattered brain regions showed both higher FA and higher diffusivity in APOE **ε2/ε3** compared to APOE **ε3/ε3**, as well as comparing APOE ε3/ε4 to APOE ε3/ε3. Only RD was decreased in small clusters in APOE ε3/ε4 compared to APOE ε3/ε3 ($P < 0.01$, cluster size = 10). And AX comparison between APOE ε2/ε3 vs. APOE ε3/ε3 showed more brain regions with higher AX in APOE ε2/ε3 carriers. MD showed similar pattern as of AX.

In addition, track-based mean FA stratified by different APOE genotype in majority of fibers demonstrated an incremental consistent pattern (44-24-33-23-34-22 chain, lowest in APOE44 and highest in APOE22 carriers); especially in right cortico-spinal tract and bilateral uncinate fasciculus (Figure 4). RD waveforms of 20 ROIs stratified by APOE genotype showed different waveforms than FA, with highest RD in APOE ε2/ε3 isoforms, and lower in APOE ε4+ carriers in all 20 ROIs. Both MD and AX measures showed very similar waveforms as of RD in 20 ROIs.

As of fMRI, 11 out of 26 seed-based fcMRI strength (mean Z-value, with $P<0.001$) stratified by different APOE genotype follow an incremental pattern with the 44-24-33-23-34-22 chain. Representative incremental mean fcMRI strength waveforms of task-positive networks seeding from intra-parietal sulcus (a), subcortical thalamus (b, c, d, e), especially the hypothalamus (f), and thalamic segment3 (d) that projected to visual cortex were demonstrated in Figure 5. On the other hand, gradual decrement of fcMRI strength with the APOE 44-24-33-23-34-22 genotypic chain of the resting-state default mode networks seeding from the posterior cingulate cortex (PCC) (g) and DMN core (h) had been observed as well (Figure 5).

3.5. fALFF and fcMRI Results

Regarding fALFF (a biomarker for functional activity), group mean image at baseline demonstrated higher fALFF pattern in cortical gray matter with only temporal cortex largely spared (Figure 6a).

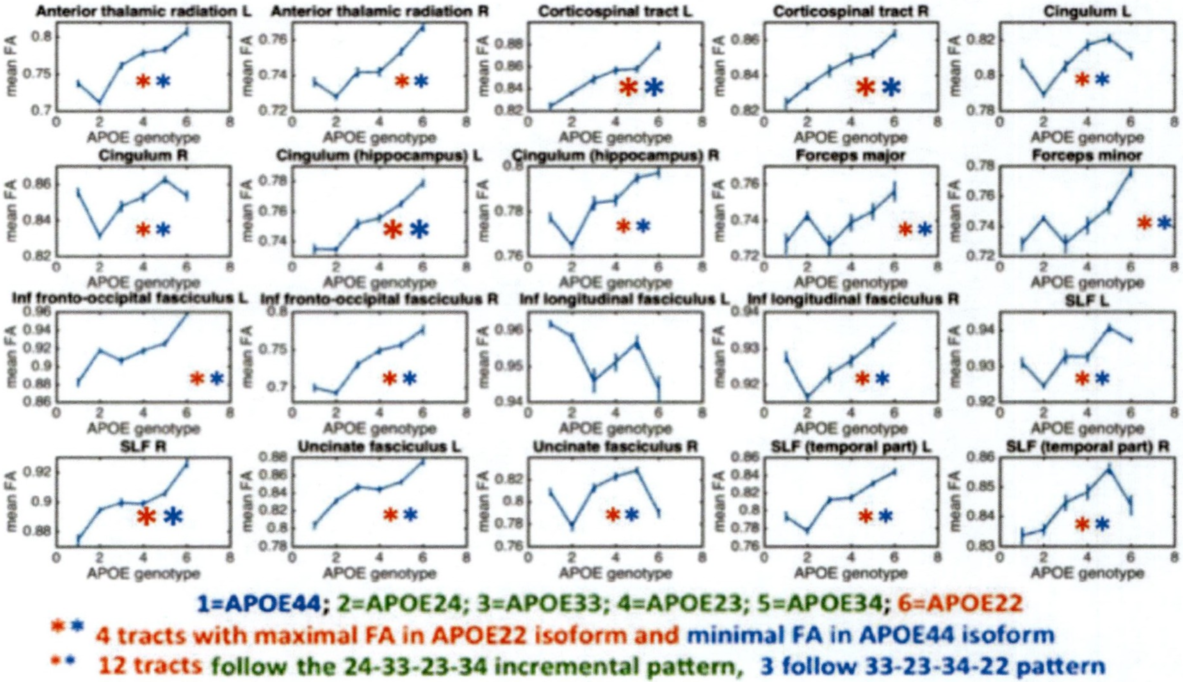

Inf = inferior; SLF = superior longitudinal fasciculus; L = left; R = right.

Figure 4. APOE genotypic effects on tract-specific mean FA in 20 brain tracts. The mean FA of bilateral corticospinal, left cingulum and right superior longitudinal fasciculus tracts (marked with large **) follow the APOE 44-24-33-23-34 incremental pattern consistently.

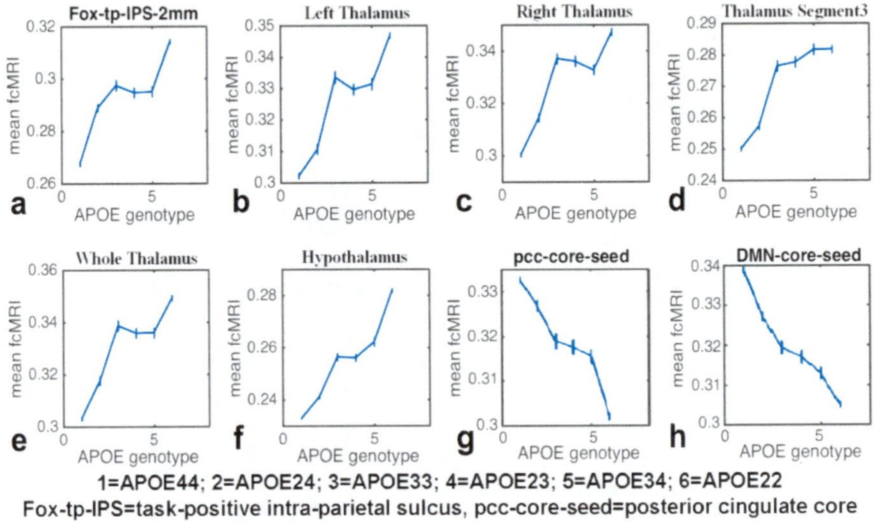

Figure 5. Effects of APOE genotype on global fcMRI strength of task-positive networks seeding from intra-parietal sulcus (a), thalamus (b,c,d,e) and hypothalamus (f) showing incremental pattern with the 44-24-33-23-34-22 chain, but detrimental pattern of resting-state default mode networks seeding from posterior cingulum (g) and core seeds of DMN (h).

Baseline aging effects demonstrated decreased activity with age in the caudate, superior middle frontal and precuneus regions, but increased activity in the cerebellum, orbito-frontal and temporal regions, as well as bilateral frontal white matter ($P < 0.001$) (Figure 6 b-c). Average fALFF activity strength over the whole brain demonstrated magnificent aging effects ($r = -0.28$, $P = 0.00001$). Average global whole-brain fALFF Z-value correlated significantly with age ($r = -0.28$, $P = 0.00002$).

Gender comparison showed slight differences with men had lower fALFF activity than women in small regions of caudate and frontal white matter clusters, but higher activity in the cerebellum (cluster corrected, $P < 0.001$) (Figure 6 d-e). Longitudinal comparison of baseline fALFF and three years follow-ups indicated decreased fALFF strength in the right inferior parietal lobe and right occipital cortex; accompanied by increased strength in the front eye field, left superior frontal and left temporal cortices ($P < 0.01$).

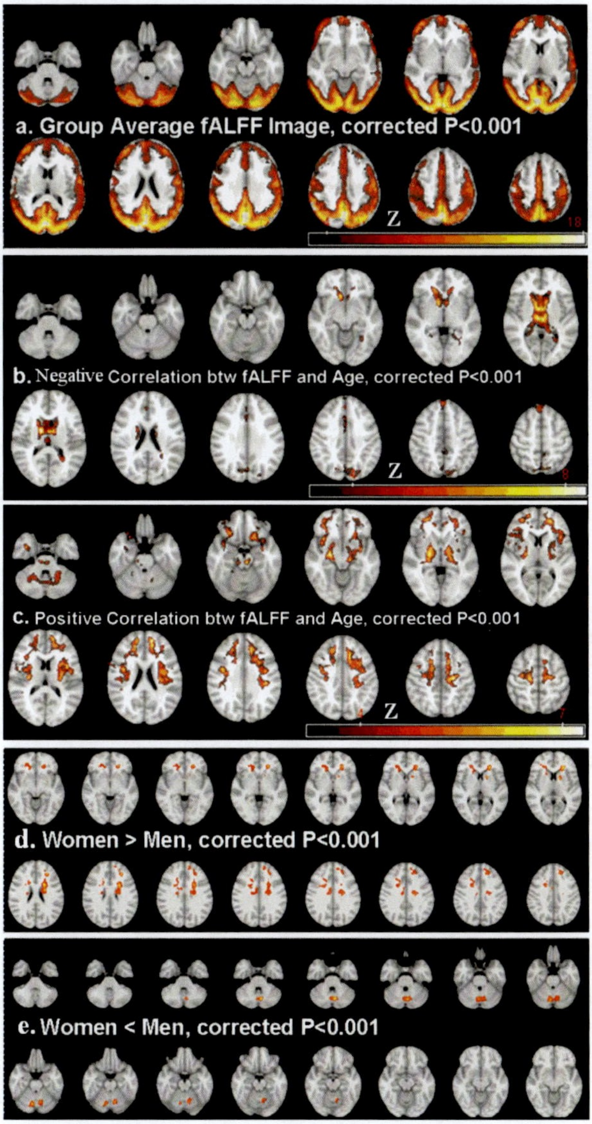

Figure 6. Functional activity measured with fALFF with group mean in a (corrected P < 0.001) showing higher fALFF in cortical gray matter with only temporal cortex largely spared. Decreased activity with age in the superior middle frontal and precuneus as well as in the cortical caudate region (b), but increased activity in the orbito-frontal and temporal regions, cerebellum and bilateral frontal white matter (c) (both cluster corrected P < 0.001) were observed. Women group had higher fALFF Z values in frontal white matter area and small regions in caudate (d) compared to men, but lower fALFF in the cerebellum (e) (both corrected P < 0.001).

3.6. Neurocognitive Tests and Correlations

For the neurocognitive tests, LME model performed to available 52 neurocognitive tests at baseline also exhibited significant aging effects ($P < 0.00001$) in almost all the test domains with worsening cognitive function at age. And similar longitudinal interval effect with significantly worse cognitive function and performance was found at a less significant level for each cognitive test at follow-up visits (most $P < 0.001$).

Significant correlations between average Z-value of fcMRI strength in the DMN and neurocognitive tests were found as following: 1. between DMN Z and digital span test (DST) total score ($r = 0.19$, $P < 0.00001$); 2. between average DMN Z and Pegboard dominant (Dom) motor function score ($r = 0.22$, $P < 0.00001$); 3. between average DMN Z and Pegboard non-dominant (NonDom) test mean score ($r = 0.17$, $P = 0.00002$); 4. between average DMN Z and category fluency (FluenCat) test mean score ($r = 0.12$, $P = 0.003$). Interestingly, significant correlations between average DMN Z and graph-theory based resting-state functional network small-worldness properties were found as well, including: 1. between DMN Z and relative local efficiency ($r = 0.15$, $P = 0.0002$); 2. between DMN Z and absolute local efficiency ($r = 0.17$, $P = 0.00002$); 3. between DMN Z and relative global efficiency ($r = 0.09$, $P = 0.02$); 4. between DMN Z and absolute global efficiency ($r = 0.1$, $P = 0.01$); and 5. between DMN Z and small-worldness configuration factor ($r = 0.15$, $P = 0.0001$). Significant correlations between age and average DMN Z ($r = -0.20$, $P < 0.00001$; $N = 608$) are noted additionally.

Significant correlations between four DTI metrics (FA/MD/AX/MD) and neurocognitive functions were found including California verbal learning test (CVLT), Fluencat, Benton visual retention total errors (BVTOT), Dom and NDom tests that measure visual perception and memory function, language fluency, communication and social function, speed and accuracy, cognitive flexibility, visual attention, spatial orientation, working memory and executive function, as well as movement speed and motor function (most $P < 0.0001$). And correlations were found consistently in all 20 tracts that connect to the whole brain, indicating both regional and global-wise associations between brain structure connectivity and neurocognitive functions.

Significant correlations among multiple imaging metrics were found as well, including: 1. average fALFF Z and mean FA of whole brain ($r = 0.26$, $P = 0.00007$); 2. average DMN Z and mean FA of whole brain ($r = 0.18$, $P = 0.007$); and 3. average DMN Z and mean FA of DMN regions ($r = 0.19$, $P = 0.004$).

4. DISCUSSIONS AND CONCLUSION

One of the main findings of DTI was the decreased FA but increased RD along the age based on both voxel-wise and track-specific analyses at both baseline and longitudinal follow-up visits. Longitudinal data revealed similar rate of change of DTI metrics associated with age and gender as to baseline results, indicating these changes were observable over a very short period (e.g., longitudinal interval of 1-3 years). Especially the significant decreases of FA along the age were consistent in most of brain regions, suggesting that microstructural white matter integrity deteriorates with age prominently and homogeneously across whole brain. RD increased with age in the regions that play important roles in memory, visual and motor function such as bilateral thalamic radiations, bilateral somatosensory cortex, visual cortex, anterior and posterior cingulate gyri, middle temporal cortex and hippocampus ($P < 0.01$, cluster size = 10). Our results suggested possible demyelination process that resulted in radial space increases in these brain tracts with age. FA/RD findings were also confirmed with significantly reduced fiber-bundles from fornix and parahippocampus at aging, as well as the latest maturation age of the cingulum bundle that was more vulnerable to demyelination and retrograde degeneration with age (Zhou 2016). While changes in AX and MD were in two-way: increased AX and MD in some tracts and cortical regions including bilateral thalamic radiation and cingulum bundles, together with decreased AX and MD in some long-distance fasciculus including bilateral cortico-spinal tract, inferior longitudinal fasciculus and optic radiation. Lower FA and higher RD indicating axonal degeneration had been found in a small sample with similar age range (Bender and Raz 2015; Kodiweera et al. 2016). A few long commissure and association fibers including corpus callosum, cortico-spinal tract, cingulum bundle and superior longitudinal fibers might also undergo Wallerian degeneration with increased RD but decreased AX along the age.

Consistent with the current view of neuroplasticity, neuroprotective and compensation roles of fMRI connectivity and activation (Scheinost et al. 2015; Trachtenberg et al. 2012; Shu et al. 2016), mean fcMRI values from resting-state DMN core and PCC core were lowest in the least risky APOE22 isoform, but highest in the most risky APOE44 isoform. However, for the task-positive networks seeding from subcortical regions including thalamus and hypothalamus seeds as well as intra-parietal sulcus, the fcMRI increases from the expected most risky to least risky genetic isoforms. These changes of divergent waveforms of fcMRI from DMN and subcortical regions had also confirmed the opposite directions of resting-state DMN network and task-positive or attentional-recruitment networks, and might indicate less efficient or over-recruitment of neuronal source utilization at most risky APOE44 carriers (Buckner et al. 2004; Sala-Llonch et al. 2015; Legon et al. 2016). On the other hand, the DTI metric of FA from majority of fibers demonstrated an incremental consistent pattern from APOE44 to APOE22 carriers, indicating micro-structural integrity was associated positively and tightly with the genotypic functional role of each APOE allele.

Associations between DMN functional connectivity and neurocognitive scores of memory, motor coordination and language social function are expected given the importance of DMN in these domains (Raichle et al. 2001; Buckner et al. 2005; Jones et al. 2011). DMN also represents more global integration function based on the significant correlations between DMN fcMRI and local/global efficiencies of network analysis (Fjell et al. 2016; Kennedy et al. 2015). Significant correlations were also found between global FA and global functional activity from fALFF; as well as between DMN fcMRI and mean FAs of the DMN region and global whole-brain. Our results of significant correlations among multiple imaging quantifications as well as with neurocognitive tests indicate neuronal degeneration, functional disconnectivity as well as white matter deterioration (demyelination, axonal and Wallerian degeneration) at age go parallel with each other, and present together with neurocognitive dysfunction (especially in the domains of memory, cognitive flexibility, visual perception and attention, as well as executive function).

Baseline aging effects found decreased fALFF functional activity in caudate and small frontal regions with aging, together with increased compensation in the frontal/temporal areas and cerebellum. Gender comparison found higher frontal fALFF but lower cerebellar functional activity in women than men. Scattered longitudinal changes and gender differences of fALFF were found with different patterns from fcMRI. Namely, decreased longitudinal fALFF in small regions of inferior parietal and occipital cortices accompanied by increased fALFF compensation in the superior frontal and temporal regions as well as cerebellum, in contrast to the largely decreased DMN but increased DAN of longitudinal fcMRI. The difference might come from the fact that the spatial distribution pattern of functional activity measured with fALFF was mainly in cortical gray matter and significantly higher in occipital, parietal and frontal cortices but with relatively lower activation pattern in temporal cortex. And fALFF measures local regional functional activity, while fcMRI measures between-regional connectivity. Although fALFF might lack of functional and spatial specialization at resting state, it had been used in epoch-related task fMRI study to reflect neuronal activation under challenged conditions (Zhou et al. 2014). It had been reported that task-based fMRI data could reflect specific cognitive function such as learning and memory, reward anticipatory and motivation, neuroplasticity and attention, social and communication skills, we expect stronger associations could be found between task-fMRI data and neurocognitive scores in extra cognitive domains (Tsvetanov et al. 2016; Bilgel et al. 2015; Worthy et al. 2015).

While our results are consistent with several published articles and are also in agreement with functional and structural connectivity findings (Westlye et al. 2012; Ward et al. 2015; Zhou et al. 2010; Trachtenberg et al. 2012), current study is still limited to the scope of conventional fMRI and DTI sequence with normal aging samples. Further improvement of the technique with acceleration-based fMRI acquisition, multi-shell and multi-b value DTI connectom based on higher-order statistical modeling and computation (Lamar et al. 2014) will be considered. And validation of our observations using other molecular imaging findings such as amyloid and tau imaging that provide pathological evidence besides the current neuroimaging findings will be explored (Scholl et al. 21016; Sheline et al. 2010).

In conclusion, different sensitivities of DTI metrics in various brain regions have been observed of the age, gender and genotypic effects. For instance, FA measures showed age effects on white matter integrity across adulthood, with increases in FA through the 30's and 40's and subsequent decreases in middle age and elderly adults. Accompanying the decreases of FA along the age in most of brain regions were the radial diffusivity increases, indicating demyelination process with age. AX and MD showed both lower and higher with age in different brain regions, suggesting possible axonal and Wallerian degenerations in these brain regions. Longitudinal regional changes in both DTI and fcMRI were similar to those demonstrating baseline effects of age, but at less significant levels. For instance decreased fcMRI in DMN but increased fcMRI in anti-correlated DAN networks were observed at both baseline and longitudinal changes. The APOE genotypic signatures of FA and functional connectivity suggested possible tight associations between myelin/neuronal activation and APOE gene, indicating different roles of APOE alleles on brain structural conductivity, demyelination and neuroplasticity. Significant correlations between neuroimaging metrics and neurocognitive tests including memory and attention were observed. Taken together, our neuroimaging and correlational neurocognitive results indicate significant and consistent age, gender and APOE genotypic effects on structural and functional connectivity at both baseline and longitudinal short-interval ranges.

REFERENCES

[1] Agosta F, Dalla Libera D, Spinelli EG, et al. Myeloid microvesicles in cerebrospinal fluid are associated with myelin damage and neuronal loss in mild cognitive impairment and Alzheimer disease. *Annals of neurology*. 2014; 76:813-825.

[2] Andrews-Hanna JR, Reidler JS, Sepulcre J, Poulin R, Buckner RL. 2010. Functional-anatomic fractionation of the brain's default network. *Neuron* 65:550-562.

[3] Bartzokis G. Age-related myelin breakdown: a developmental model of cognitive decline and Alzheimer's disease. *Neurobiology of aging*. 2004; 25:5-18; author reply 49-62.

[4] Basser PJ. Inferring microstructural features and the physiological state of tissues from diffusion-weighted images. *NMR in biomedicine*. 1995; 8:333-344.

[5] Bender AR and Raz N. Normal-appearing cerebral white matter in healthy adults: mean change over 2 years and individual differences in change. *Neurobiology of aging*. 2015; 36:1834-1848.

[6] Bendfeldt K, Kuster P, Traud S, Egger H, Winklhofer S, Mueller-Lenke N, Naegelin Y, Gass A, Kappos L, Matthews PM, Nichols TE, Radue EW, Borgwardt SJ. Association of regional gray matter volume loss and progression of white matter lesions in multiple sclerosis - A longitudinal voxel-based morphometry study. *Neuroimage*. 2009; 45:60-67.

[7] Bilgel M, An Y, Zhou Y, et al. Individual estimates of age at detectable amyloid onset for risk factor assessment. Alzheimer's & dementia: *The journal of the Alzheimer's Association* 2015; 36(8): 2333.

[8] Billiet T, Vandenbulcke M, Madler B, et al. Age-related microstructural differences quantified using myelin water imaging and advanced diffusion MRI. *Neurobiology of aging*. 2015; 36:2107-2121.

[9] Bjartmar C, Wujek JR, Trapp BD. Axonal loss in the pathology of MS: consequences for understanding the progressive phase of the disease. *J Neurol Sci*. 2003; 206:165-171.

[10] Bodini B, Khaleeli Z, Cercignani M, Miller DH, Thompson AJ, Ciccarelli O. Exploring the relationship between white matter and gray matter damage in early primary progressive multiple sclerosis: an in vivo study with TBSS and VBM. *Hum Brain Mapp*. 2009; 30:2852-2861.

[11] Buckner RL, Snyder AZ, Shannon BJ, LaRossa G, Sachs R, Fotenos AF, Sheline YI, Klunk WE, Mathis CA, Morris JC, Mintun MA. Molecular, structural, and functional characteri-zation of Alzheimer's disease: evidence for a relationship between default activity, amyloid, and memory. *J Neurosci*. 2005; 25:7709-7717.

[12] Buckner RL. Memory and executive function in aging and AD: multiple factors that cause decline and reserve factors that compensate. *Neuron*. 2004; 44:195-208.

[13] Fjell AM, Sneve MH, Storsve AB, Grydeland H, Yendiki A, Walhovd KB. Brain Events Underlying Episodic Memory Changes in Aging: A Longitudinal Investigation of Structural and Functional Connectivity. *Cereb Cortex*. 2016; 26:1272-1286.

[14] Forn C, Barros-Loscertales A, Escudero J, Benlloch V, Campos S, Antonia Parcet M, Avila C. Compensatory activations in patients with multiple sclerosis during preserved performance on the auditory N-back task. *Hum Brain Mapp*. 2007; 28:424-430.

[15] Fox MD and Raichle ME. Spontaneous fluctuations in brain activity observed with functional magnetic resonance imaging. *Nat Rev Neurosci*. 2007; 8:700-711.

[16] Gazes Y, Bowman FD, Razlighi QR, O'Shea D, Stern Y, Habeck C. White matter tract covariance patterns predict age-declining cognitive abilities. *NeuroImage*. 2016; 125:53-60.

[17] Goh JO, An Y, Resnick SM. Differential trajectories of age-related changes in components of executive and memory processes. *Psychol Aging*. 2012; 27:707-719.

[18] Horch RA, Gore JC, Does MD. Origins of the ultrashort-T2 1H NMR signals in myelinated nerve: a direct measure of myelin content? *Magnetic resonance in medicine*. 2011; 66:24-31.

[19] Hudak, A., Warner, M., Marquez de la Plata, C., Moore, C., Harper, C. & Diaz-Arrastia, R. Brain morphometry changes and depressive symptoms after traumatic brain injury. *Psychiatry Res*. 2011; 191(3): 160–165.

[20] Huster D, Yao X, Hong M. Membrane protein topology probed by (1)H spin diffusion from lipids using solid-state NMR spectroscopy. *Journal of the American Chemical Society*. 2002; 124:874-883.

[21] Jones, DT et al. Age-related changes in the default mode network are more advanced in Alzheimer disease. *Neurology*. 2011; 77:1524-1531, doi:10.1212/WNL.0b013e318233b33d.

[22] Kennedy KM, Rodrigue KM, Bischof GN, Hebrank AC, Reuter-Lorenz PA, Park DC. Age trajectories of functional activation under conditions of low and high processing demands: an adult lifespan fMRI study of the aging brain. *Neuroimage*. 2015; 104:21-34.

[23] Kochunov P, Glahn DC, Lancaster J, et al. Fractional anisotropy of cerebral white matter and thickness of cortical gray matter across the lifespan. *NeuroImage*. 2011; 58:41-49.

[24] Kodiweera C, Alexander AL, Harezlak J, McAllister TW, Wu YC. Age effects and gender differences in human brain white matter of young to middle-aged adults: A DTI, NODDI, and q-space study. *NeuroImage*. 2016; 128:180-192.

[25] Kolasa M, Hakulinen U, Helminen M, Hagman S, Raunio M, Rossi M, Brander A, Dastidar P, Elovaara. Longitudinal assessment of clinically isolated syndrome with diffusion tensor imaging and volumetric MRI. *Clin Imaging I.* 2015; 39:207-212.

[26] Lamar M, Zhou XJ, Charlton RA, Dean D, Little D, Deoni. In vivo quantification of white matter microstructure for use in aging: a focus on two emerging techniques. *Am J Geriatr Psychiatry*. 2014; 22(2):111-121.

[27] Legon W, Punzell S, Dowlati E, Adams SE, Stiles AB, Moran RJ. Altered Prefrontal Excitation/Inhibition Balance and Prefrontal Output: Markers of Aging in Human Memory Networks. *Cereb Cortex.* 2016; 26(11):4315-4326.

[28] Lisak RP. Neurodegeneration in multiple sclerosis: defining the problem. *Neurology*. 2007; 68:S5-12; discussion S43-54.

[29] Lowe MJ, Beall EB, Sakaie KE, Koenig KA, Stone L, Marrie RA, Phillips MD Resting state sensorimotor functional connectivity in multiple sclerosis inversely correlates with transcallosal motor

pathway transverse diffusivity. *Hum Brain Mapp*. 2008; 29:818-827.

[30] McCarrey AC, An Y, Kitner-Triolo MH, Ferrucci L, Resnick SM. Gender differences in cognitive trajectories in clinically normal older adults. *Psychology and aging*. 2016; 31:166-175.

[31] Raichle ME, MacLeod AM, Snyder AZ, Powers WJ, Gusnard DA, Shulman GL. A default mode of brain function. *Proc Natl Acad Sci* U S A. 2001; 98:676-682.

[32] Rocca MA, Preziosa P, Mesaros S, Pagani E, Dackovic J, Stosic-Opincal T, Drulovic J, Filippi M. Clinically Isolated Syndrome Suggestive of Multiple Sclerosis: Dynamic Patterns of Gray and White Matter Changes-A 2-year MR Imaging Study. *Radiology*. 2016; 278:841-853.

[33] Sala-Llonch R, Bartres-Faz D, Junque C. Reorganization of brain networks in aging: a review of functional connectivity studies. *Front Psychol*. 2015; 6:663.

[34] Sasson E, Doniger GM, Pasternak O, Tarrasch R, Assaf Y. Structural correlates of cognitive domains in normal aging with diffusion tensor imaging. *Brain structure & function*. 2012; 217:503-515.

[35] Scheinost D, Finn ES, Tokoglu F, et al. Gender differences in normal age trajectories of functional brain networks. *Hum Brain Mapp*. 2015; 36:1524-1535.

[36] Scholl M, Lockhart SN, Schonhaut DR et al. PET Imaging of Tau Deposition in the Aging Human Brain. *Neuron*. 2016; 89(5):971-982.

[37] Sheline YI, Raichle ME, Snyder AZ, et al. Amyloid plaques disrupt resting state default mode network connectivity in cognitively normal elderly. *Biological psychiatry*. 2010; 67:584-587.

[38] Shu, H, et al. Opposite Neural Trajectories of Apolipoprotein E 4 and 2 Alleles with Aging Associated with Different Risks of Alzheimer's Disease. *Cereb Cortex*. 2016; 26:1421-1429.

[39] Thiessen JD, Zhang Y, Zhang H, et al. Quantitative MRI and ultrastructural examination of the cuprizone mouse model of demyelination. *NMR in biomedicine*. 2013; 26:1562-1581.

[40] Trachtenberg AJ, Filippini N, Ebmeier KP, Smith SM, Karpe F, Mackay CE. The effects of APOE on the functional architecture of the resting brain. *NeuroImage*. 2012; 59:565-572.

[41] Trachtenberg AJ, Filippini N, Ebmeier KP, Smith SM, Karpe F, Mackay CE. The effects of APOE on the functional architecture of the resting brain. *NeuroImage*. 2012; 59:565-572.

[42] Tsvetanov KA, Henson RN, Tyler LK, Razi A, Geerligs L, Ham TE, Rowe JB, Cambridge Centre for A, Neuroscience. Extrinsic and Intrinsic Brain Network Connectivity Maintains Cognition across the Lifespan Despite Accelerated Decay of Regional Brain Activation. *J Neurosci*. 2016; 36:3115-3126.

[43] Ward AM, Mormino EC, Huijbers W, Schultz AP, Hedden T, Sperling RA. Relationships between default-mode network connectivity, medial temporal lobe structure, and age-related memory deficits. *Neurobiology of aging*. 2015; 36:265-272.

[44] Westlye LT, Reinvang I, Rootwelt H, Espeseth T. Effects of APOE on brain white matter microstructure in healthy adults. *Neurology* 2012; 79:1961-1969.

[45] Worthy DA, Davis T, Gorlick MA, Cooper JA, Bakkour A, Mumford JA, Poldrack RA, Todd Maddox W. Neural correlates of state-based decision-making in younger and older adults. *Neuroimage*. 2015; 130:13-23.

[46] Yount, R., Raschke, KA, Biru, M, et al. Traumatic brain injury and atrophy of the cingulate gyrus. *J Neuropsychiatry Clin Neurosci*. 2002; 14(4): 416–423.

[47] Zhou J, Greicius MD, Gennatas ED, et al. Divergent network connectivity changes in behavioural variant frontotemporal dementia and Alzheimer's disease. Brain: *A journal of neurology*. 2010;133:1352-1367.

[48] Zhou XJ. Diffusion tensor imaging: techniques and clinical applications. *Conference proceedings: Annual International Conference of the IEEE Engineering in Medicine and Biology Society*. 2004; 7:5223-5225.

[49] Zhou Y, Lui YW, Zuo XN, Milham MP, Reaume J, Grossman RI, Ge Y. 2014. Characterization of thalamo-cortical association using amplitude and connectivity of functional MRI in mild traumatic brain injury. *J Magn Reson Imaging* 39:1558-1568.

[50] Zhou Y, Milham MP, Lui YW, Miles L, Reaume J, Sodickson DK, Grossman RI, Ge Y. Default-mode network disruption in mild traumatic brain injury. *Radiology*. 2002; 265:882-892.

[51] Zhou Y. Abnormal structural and functional hypothalamic connectivity in mild traumatic brain injury. *J Magn Reson Imaging*. 2017; 45:1105-1112.

[52] Zhou Y. *Functional Neuroimaging with Multiple Modalities*. Nova Publishers. 2016.

[53] Zhou Y. *Neuroimaging in Mild Traumatic Brain Injury*. Nova Publishers. 2017a.

[54] Zhou Y. *Neuroimaging in Multiple Sclerosis*. Nova Publishers. 2017b.

[55] Zhou Y. *Functional Neuroimaging Methods and Frontiers*. Nova Publishers. 2018.

Chapter 3

LONGITUDINAL EFFECTS OF AGE AND SMOKING ON ENDOTHELIAL FUNCTION ASSESSED BY QUANTITATIVE MRI

ABSTRACT

Our previous baseline results suggested that newly developed MRI biomarkers of endothelial dysfunction (EDF) were sensitive to both age and smoking effects that act independently and similarly. The purpose of this study is to assess various surrogates of EDF at 18-month follow-up compared to baseline in smokers and older subjects. Measures of peripheral vascular reactivity were assessed via dynamic venous susceptometry and oximetry, arterial velocimetry and multi-segment pulse-wave velocity (PWV) of thoracic and abdominal aorta in the form of an integrated protocol with a time-resolved multi-echo gradient-recalled echo (GRE) sequence. Total 113 subjects out of 169 baseline participants finished 18-month 2nd visits consisted of 39 young non-smokers, 14 young smokers, 30 old non-smokers and 30 old smokers.. Vascular reactivity was evaluated following cuff-induced hyperemia via time-resolved blood flow velocity and venous saturation of oxygen (SvO_2) in the femoral artery and vein, respectively, by quantifying post-occlusion change relative to baseline values. Velocimetry-based arterial parameters included pulse ratio, hyperemic index and forward flow time. PWV was assessed in aortic arch, thoracoabdominal aorta and iliofemoral arteries. Two-way ANOVA indicated that there was no interaction between smoking and age ($P = 0.09$-0.78) for all parameters evaluated at follow-up visits. Paired t-test for the same MRI parameter between two visits across all subjects showed significant longitudinal worsening in several parameters including reduced overshoot ($P = 0.003$) and arterial hyperemic index ($P < 0.0001$), as well as increased pulse ratio ($P < 0.0001$) and iliofemoral PWV (ifPWV) ($P = 0.0008$) at 2nd visit compared to 1st visit. The mean of fractional variation of test-retest to the longitudinal variation was 32%, suggesting data variation does not contribute significantly to the longitudinal observations. Strong correlations were observed in the same parameters measured at both visits including washout time, upslope, overshoot, forward flow time T_{ff}, thoracoabdominal, iliofemoral and total PWVs (all with $r > 0.4$, $P < 0.01$). Correlational analysis among parameters between 1st visit and 2nd visits showed significant influences ($r > 0.29$, $P < 0.05$) of the small venous reactivity parameters (i.e., washout, upslope and overshoot) at 1st visit on the arterial stiffness parameters (aortic arch, thoracoabdominal and iliofemoral PWVs) at follow-ups. Significant correlations between MRI parameters and cardiovascular risk factors were found ($|r| > 0.2$, $P < 0.05$) at longitudinal follow-up visit, as well as between cardiovascular risk factors at 1st visit and MRI parameters at 2nd visit. In conclusion, the vascular reactivity parameters in this study demonstrated significantly worsening of microvascular circulation and arterial stiffness with age and in smokers at 18-month follow-ups. These alterations are more likely to be resulted from atherosclerosis and cardiovascular risk increments over time in especially smokers and elderly people.

1. Introduction

Based on Framingham heart study, the hazard ratio of smoking ranked 2nd, next to diabetes, among all the cardiovascular disease (CVD) risk factors (Pencina et al. 2009). A healthy endothelium is a key player in the maintenance of vascular health and proper function. Endothelial dysfunction (EDF) is an early event in atherogenesis (Davignon and Ganz 2004), characterized by a reduction in the availability of nitric oxide (NO) that would lead to increased inflammation, improper vasodilation, and thrombosis (Ambroe and Barua 2004). NO can be reduced and consumed by reactive oxygen species (ROS) such as superoxide and peroxynitirite due to impaired bioavailability (Cooke and Dzau 1997). Cigarette smoking, which has been estimated to produce over 4,000 known and over 100,000 unknown ROS constituents (Church 1986; WHO 2011), could damage the endothelium and initiate intima-media thickening (IMT) by causing a ROS-induced NO reduction. It has been shown that smoking as few as two cigarettes per day doubles the number of damaged circulating endothelial cell (Hamburg 2011; Corretti et al. 2002). EDF is believed to be the earliest initiator of atherogenesis followed by the well-known sequelae leading to neurovascular and heart diseases (Celermajer et al. 1994). Various conditions such as hypertension, hypercholesterolemia, diabetes mellitus as well as age could lead to lower NO release, ROS generation and EDF (Kiowski et al. 1994; Hallden et al. 2013).

Our previous imaging findings at baseline demonstrated that various MRI biomarkers of EDF were sensitive to both age and smoking effects that act independently and similarly (Langham et al. 2015). Implementing a relatively new MRI multi-echo gradient-recalled echo (GRE) sequence in a previous large cohort study, central and peripheral vascular reactivities were measured with a safe blood pressure cuff (i.e., cuff paradigm) to the upper right thigh, mimicking ischemia condition. The peripheral vascular reactivity (VR) metrics including pulse wave velocity (PWV) of the aorta, iliac and femoral circulation were incorporated into a single examination protocol for dynamic venous oximetry that makes use of venous oxygen saturation as an endogenous tracer (Langham et al. 2009; Langham et al. 2011). Central cerebral VR (CVR) and EDF were quantified with both phase and magnitude-based MRI sequences (Zhou 2017). Specifically, we found aging effects among non-smokers; for instance, older non-smokers (ONS) had lower upslope (−22.7%, $P < 0.01$) and overshoot (−29.4%, $P < 0.01$), but elevated baseline pulse ratio (+14.9%, $P < 0.01$) as well as central and peripheral PWV (all $P < 0.05$) compared to young non-smokers (YNS). Regarding smoking effects, in young group, relative to YNS, young smokers (YS) had lower upslope (−23.6%, $P < 0.01$) and longer washout time (13.5%, $P < 0.05$). In old-aged group, old smokers (OS) had lower upslope (−33.0%, $P < 0.01$) compared to ONS (Langham et al. 2015). Using breath-holding index (BHI) measured with fast brain imaging sequence to the brain, we also reported significantly lower neurovascular reactivity (NVR) ($P \leq 0.01$) based on velocimetry in smokers and especially elderly smokers compared to young and non-smoking subjects. Marginally smoking effect was observed between smokers and non-smokers ($P = 0.05$ for slope and $P = 0.05$ for BHI) based on magnitude method (Zhou 2017).

Significantly lower cerebral blood flow (CBF) values were also present with age in all brain regions, especially at cortical and sub-cortical gray matter regions ($P < 0.01$, cluster corrected) (Zhou 2017). And regionally higher CBF was observed in the subcortical putamen, thalamus and posterior cingulate regions in women than in men. Furthermore, longitudinal interval effects showed CBF decrement in frontal, temporal, posterior cingulate, and caudate regions, accompanied with CBF increment compensation in subcortical putamen and pallidum as well as cerebellar regions at ~4 years follow-up visits. And we had found distinct and independent voxel-wise brain CBF changes identified from several methods, with prominent effects of age and longitudinal changes (in relatively old participants) compared to other factors including gender, APOE, amyloid load and physiological challenges (Zhou 2017).

Functional imaging reflects largely real-time neural activity, intertwined neural circuits plasticity and compensation, thus could be used to test reversible risk factors (Harris 2004). The purpose of this study is to evaluate the longitudinal changes as well as scan repeatability. Our assumptions are: longitudinal EDF alterations in the whole body will be observed both in elderly participants and smokers at 2nd visit; and the test-retest variability will not contribute significantly to the observed quantifications. In order to assess various surrogates of EDF at 18-month follow-up compared to baseline, the integrated MRI protocol were performed in 169 baseline, 21 test-retest and 113 longitudinal scans Data consistency was evaluated with repeatability and ANOVA, and correlational causality analyses as well as longitudinal analyses were performed to MRI metrics and cardiovascular risk factors at two visits. We expect significant aging and smoking effects of these parameters at both visits, and worsening of these parameters, especially over 18 month period in both non-smokers and smokers sub-groups.

2. METHODS

2.1. Subjects

169 baseline participants, 113 follow-ups during approximately 18 months from the initial visit and 21 within-one-month repeatability studies at follow-up visits were performed. The 2nd-visit follow-up subjects were divided into four sub-groups: 39 young healthy non-smokers (YNS; age = 31.5 ± 0.8, age range: 26–40 years), 14 young smokers (YS; 36.1 ± 0.8 years), 30 old healthy non-smokers (ONS; 58.4 ± 0.6 years, age range: 51–65 years), and 30 old smokers (OS; N = 10, 57.5 ± 1.2 years). Smoking severity in terms of cigarette pack years was 6.6 ± 0.7 and 17.6 ± 3.9 for young and old smokers respectively. Demographic information of participants at baseline and 18-month follow-up visit was listed in Table 1 and Table 2 respectively. At 2nd visit, low-density cholesterol (LDL) level was significantly lower in the OS than ONS (P = 0.007), and higher LDL as well as total cholesterol levels were observed in the ONS than YNS groups. C-reactive protein (CRP) level was significantly lower in OS than ONS (P = 0.01), but significantly higher in ONS than YNS ($P<0.05$). Significantly higher body mass index (BMI) in OS compared to ONS as well as higher BMI

in ONS compared to YNS ($P = 0.01$) were found at 2nd visit. Since only partial participants enrolled in the 2nd visits due to unavailability and other reasons, a few cardiovascular characteristics were not different significantly between two sub-groups at 2nd visit but indicated aging and smoking effects at 1st visit. These cardiovascular factors include: significantly lower total cholesterol and LDL levels in YNS than ONS; significantly higher high-density cholesterol (HDL) level in YNS than ONS as well as higher CRP in OS than ONS, and significantly higher systolic blood pressure (SBP) in the ONS than YNS at baseline ($P < 0.05$).

2.2. MRI Imaging

All MRI studies were performed at MRI 3T (Siemens Tim Trio) scanner with extremity and body matrix coils. The quantitative MRI protocol to evaluate central and peripheral vascular reactivity comprised measurement of reactive hyperemia in the leg induced by cuff occlusion (2 mins baseline, 5 mins occlusion and 6 mins recovery). A multi-echo GRE sequence with velocity-encoded projections and flow-compensated background suppression was launched to measure venous saturation of oxygen (SvO_2) and arterial velocity simultaneously at 1.25s/120msec temporal resolution (Langham et al. 2011). Vascular reactivity was evaluated following cuff-induced hyperemia via time-resolved blood flow velocity and SvO_2 in the femoral artery and vein, respectively. SvO_2 dynamics yielded washout time (time to minimum SvO_2), resaturation rate (upslope) and maximum change from baseline (overshoot). Arterial parameters included pulse ratio (PR), hyperemic index (HI) and duration of hyperemia or forward flow time (T_{ff}). Pulse-wave velocity (PWV) was assessed in aortic arch, thoracoabdominal aorta and iliofemoral arteries.

2.3. MRI Sequence and Data Analysis

Measures of vascular reactivity were obtained as the post-occlusion change relative to baseline values. Time-resolved blood flow velocity and SvO_2 levels were measured simultaneously in the femoral artery and vein, respectively (thereby requiring a single cuff occlusion only) (Langham et al. 2015). Briefly, lower limb ischemia was induced by applying a blood pressure cuff (SC120D model, Hokanson, Bellevue, WA, USA) to the upper right thigh. The cuff was inflated to 75 mmHg above the subject's systolic blood pressure (SBP), but not exceeding 250 mmHg. The cuff paradigm consisted of 2 minutes of baseline, 5 minutes of cuff occlusion, and 6 minutes of recovery. During the baseline (pre-occlusion) period, blood flow velocity and oxygenation were quantified successively. Ten seconds prior to cuff release the pulse sequence was launched to measure time-resolve arterial blood flow velocity and venous oxygenation simultaneously with temporal resolution of 120 ms and 1.25 s, respectively, for a period of 70 seconds.

Ungated absolute blood flow velocity was obtained utilizing a projection technique by computing the phase differences between velocity-encoded projections after isolating blood signal (Langham et al. 2010). During baseline, the velocity-encoding parameter, referred to as VENC (determining the highest velocity that can be unambiguously measured), was set to 80 cm/s and temporal resolution was 20 ms. During the post-occlusion (hyperemia) period, since the arterial velocity is significantly greater, higher VENC = 125 cm/s and 175 cm/s were selected, at a temporal resolution of 120 ms (reduction in the temporal resolution results from interleaving velocimetry and oximetry). The fractional blood oxygenation level (%HbO_2) in the femoral vein was estimated by field mapping, yielding the magnetic susceptibility difference between intravascular blood and surrounding tissue.

Central and peripheral regional pulse-wave velocities were quantified in the same imaging session following the cuff protocol. The protocol starts with acquisition of a series of oblique sagittal slices for visualizing the ascending and descending aorta. Multiple axial slices are then acquired below the pulmonary trunk to image both ascending and proximal descending aorta in the same imaging plane. Subsequently, a suitable slice and readout direction are selected for the ungated acquisition of velocity-encoded projections at a temporal resolution of 7.4 ms for about 12 sec to cover 10-12 cardiac cycles. VENC of 180 cm/s was chosen, thereby ensuring accurate mapping of the velocity-time curve with complex difference intensity at the "foot" of the systolic upstroke, which is needed to determine the pulse pressure transit time via "foot-to-foot" method (Laurent et al. 2006).

Thoracoabdominal aorta and iliofemoral PWVs were obtained analogously except that the velocity-encoded projections were collected simultaneously at two slice locations. For thoracoabdominal aortic PWV measurement, velocity-encoded projections were collected at a proximal location of the descending aorta as well as distally in the abdominal aorta (superior to the iliac bifurcation). Finally, for the peripheral iliofemoral PWV, the coils were positioned over the abdomen and upper thighs to enable simultaneous acquisition of projections at a slice inferior to the iliac bifurcation and a slice superior to the popliteal artery. The slightly lower temporal resolution of 12 ms was compensated by the greater path length of the pulse pressure wave, therefore yielding similar precision at this site. VENC values were 125 cm/s for thoracoabdominal aorta and 75 cm/s for iliofemoral arteries, respectively, to optimize the complex difference signal intensity (Bernstein et al. 2004).

2.4. MRI Vascular Reactivity Parameter Quantification

2.4.1. Quantification of Time-Resolved blood flow velocity *in the Femoral Vein*

First, Baseline (i.e. pre-occlusion) velocities were averaged over multiple heart beats (typically 6–8 beats), yielding peak-systolic velocity (Vs), peak retrograde velocity (Vr), and peak late antegrade velocity (Va). From these parameters the *pulse ratio (PR),* defined as the ratio of systolic and diastolic pulsatility, (Vs- Vr)/(Va-Vr), was derived. Parameters related to hyperemia condition included *time of forward flow* (T_{ff}), and *hyperemic index (HI)* defined as the ratio of hyperemic peak flow velocity (Vmax) to (Va-Vr).

2.4.1. Quantification of Time-Resolved SvO_2 *in the Femoral Vein*

To quantify venous oxygenation level, magnetic field inhomogeneity was corrected to remove large-scale static field inhomogeneity (Fernandez-Seara et al. 2006). Subsequently, SvO_2 was computed from the phase differences between the femoral vein and artery, incorporating individual hematocrit level determined from blood sample. The femoral artery, located adjacent to the femoral vein, was chosen to minimize observer-dependent selection of a reference region. The SvO_2 dynamic time-course curve was parameterized yielding *washout time*, *upslope* and *overshoot (OS)*. The washout time is the time elapsed to observe the oxygen-depleted capillary blood at the imaging slice after cuff deflation at t = 0 s. Upslope and overshoot are defined as the mean resaturation rate during hyperemia and the subsequent maximal above-baseline SvO_2 level, respectively.

2.4.2. Pulse-Wave Velocity Quantification

The complex difference intensity signals from proximal and distal slices were spatially averaged along the readout direction within the vessel boundary for each time point (temporal resolution = 7.4 ms for *aortic arch PWV (aPWV)* and 12ms for thoracoabdominal *PWV (daPWV)* and iliofemoral PWVs *(ifPWV)*. The time courses from proximal and distal locations were then plotted jointly to determine the propagation time of the wave-front (Langham et al. 2011). Estimation of the wave-front propagation time is equivalent to the foot-to-foot technique commonly utilized in tonometric studies (Wikinson et al. 1998). This measurement was performed for each heart beat and averaged over all cardiac cycles.

For all arterial segments, PWV was calculated as: PWV = L/Δt, where L is the path length of the pressure wave between measurement sites, and Δt is the wave-front propagation time averaged over multiple heartbeats. For the thoracoabdominal aorta and iliofemoral artery segments, path length was determined from the anatomic axial images used for planning purposes. Specifically, the artery's centroid was manually recorded from the proximal descending aorta to the distal abdominal aorta, corresponding to the measurement locations of the velocity-encoded projections, and path length was computed as the sum of the displacement of the artery between slices. Similar for the iliofemoral segment, the path length for the iliofemoral segment was estimated the same way from the iliac bifurcation to the popliteal artery. Finally, *total PWV (tPWV)* was computed as the sum of path lengths along all three arterial segments divided by the sum of propagation times. A total of 10 MRI metrics (washout, upslope, overshot, pulse ratio-PR, forward flow time-T_{ff}, hyperemic index-HI, aortic PWV-aPWV, thoraco-abdominal PWV-daPWV and iliofemoral PWV-ifPWV) were further quantified and processed in this chapter.

2.5. Statistical Analysis

Two-way ANOVA analyses were performed to determine whether effects of smoking and age could be separated from one another. If there was no interaction between smoking and age (as found at 1st vist and as expected), one-way ANOVA was performed and followed by post-hoc analysis of the parameters between the YNS vs. YS, ONS vs. OS and YNS vs. ONS via unpaired and paired t-tests, with $p < 0.05$ being considered significant. Nonparametric Wilcoxon tests were performed in situations where parameters were not normally distributed. Further, inter-parameter correlations were performed to evaluate associations between parameters derived with different MRI methods and between vascular territories at two visits using Spearman rank and Pearson correlation methods. All analyses were performed in Excel and JMP (JMP®, Version 11, SAS Institute Inc., Cary, NC).

Table 1. Subject and cardiovascular characteristics (means ± standard error) at baseline

Groups	Y-NS (N = 45)	Y-S (N = 39)	O-NS (N = 45)	O-S (N = 40)
Age (years)	30.2 ± 0.7	32.1 ± 0.7	57.8 ± 0.6	56.3 ± 0.6
Men	17	20	13	22
White	29	16	29	14
Black	6	21	9	26
Asian	10	2	7	0
SBP (mmHg)	115.4 ± 1.9**	116.7 ± 2.2	122.7 ± 2.7**	127.3 ± 2.2
DBP (mmHg)	73.4 ± 1.2	75.3 ± 1.9	76.7 ± 1.5	81.0 ± 1.5
MAP (mmHg)	87.5 ± 1.2	89.1 ± 1.9	91.6 ± 1.8	96.4 ± 1.6
HR (bpm)	75.6 ± 1.8	75.2 ± 2.3	75.9 ± 1.3	76.9 ± 1.7
BMI (kg/m^2)	23.4 ± 0.5* **	26.1 ± 0.7*	26.2 ± 0.6**	26.5 ± 0.6
Total Chol (mg/dL)	170.5 ± 4.8**	172.7 ± 6.4	196.2 ± 5.7**	196.3 ± 6.2
LDL (mg/dL)	98.5 ± 3.7**	103.6 ± 5.6	123.0 ± 5.1**	121.4 ± 5.4
HDL (mg/dL)	57.5 ± 2.1*	48.7 ± 2.4*	55.5 ± 2.5	54.6 ± 2.4
Triglycerides (mg/dL)	70.9 ± 4.9	95.5 ± 11.1	95.3 ± 12.2	117.2 ± 14.5
CRP (mg/L)	1.3 ± 0.2	2.0 ± 0.4	1.8 ± 0.3^	4.6 ± 1.0^

MAP (mean arterial pressure), calculated as MAP = SBP/3+DBPx2/3 (SBP = systolic blood pressure, DBP = diastolic blood pressure), Chol = cholesterol, LDL = low-density cholesterol, HDL = high-density cholesterol, CRP = C-reactive protein.

^ P < 0.05, older smokers versus older non-smokers.

* P < 0.05, young non-smokers versus young smokers.

** P < 0.05, young non-smokers versus older non-smokers.

Table 2. Subject and cardiovascular characteristics (means ± standard error) at 18-month follow-up visit

Groups	Y-NS (N = 39)	Y-S (N = 14)	O-NS (N = 30)	O-S (N = 30)
Age (years)	31.5 ± 0.8	36.1 ± 0.8	58.4 ± 0.6	57.5 ± 1.2
Men	17	4	10	14
White	27	3	18	9
Black	6	9	8	21
Asian	5	1	5	0
SBP (mmHg)	115.5 ± 2.5	124.4 ± 3.1	121.4 ± 2.5	124.0 ± 3.7
DBP (mmHg)	73.8 ± 1.8	80.9 ± 2.0	77.9 ± 1.5	79.9 ± 2.8
MAP (mmHg)	87.6 ± 2.0	94.9 ± 2.3	92.4 ± 1.6	94.6 ± 2.8
HR (bpm)	75.6 ± 1.8	75.2 ± 2.3	75.9 ± 1.3	76.9 ± 1.7
BMI (kg/m^2)	23.4 ± 0.5***	27.6 ± 0.8*	26.2 ± 0.6**	26.4 ± 0.6
Total Chol (mg/dL)	171.1 ± 5.3	176.0 -	194.1 ± 5.1	161.6 ± 13.5
LDL (mg/dL)	99.4 ± 4.3	74.0 -	118.2 ± 4.7^	75.8 ± 4.8^
HDL (mg/dL)	55.8 ± 2.5	90.7 -	56.8 ± 2.9	46.4 ± 3.5
Triglycerides (mg/dL)	79.1 ± 6.5	58.0 -	96.2 ± 6.3	155.6 ± 42.7
CRP (mg/L)	1.3 ± 0.2**	0.9 -	2.0 ± 0.2^**	0.8 ± 0.2^**

MAP (mean arterial pressure), calculated as MAP = SBP/3+DBPx2/3 (SBP = systolic blood pressure, DBP = diastolic blood pressure), Chol = cholesterol, LDL = low-density cholesterol, HDL = high-density cholesterol, CRP = C-reactive protein.

^ $P < 0.05$, older smokers versus older non-smokers.

* $P < 0.05$, young non-smokers versus young smokers.

** $P < 0.05$, young non-smokers versus older non-smokers.

- indicates statistical result is not available due to relatively small number of participants.

3. Results

3.1. Data Consistency

The mean fractional variation of test-retest within 1-month to the longitudinal (18-month) variation was 32%, suggesting data variation does not contribute significantly to the longitudinal observations (Table 3). Paired t-test for the same MRI parameter for 21 sub-sample subjects found significant longitudinal worsening in several parameters including reduced overshoot (P = 0.003) and arterial hyperemic index (P < 0.0001), as well as increased pulse ratio (P < 0.0001) and iliofemoral PWV (P = 0.0008). As expected, similar temporal dynamics were observed to all MRI parameters at both initial and 18-month follow-up visits; for instance, oximetry and velocimetry generated almost the same curves at two visits for one representative non-smoker (Figure 1). Significant correlations were observed in the same parameters measured at 1st time and longitudinal follow-ups including washout time, upslope, overshoot, forward flow time (T_{ff}), thoracoabdominal PWV, iliofemoral and total PWVs (all with r > 0.4, P < 0.01). An example of significant correlation of SvO_2 overshoot between two visits (r = 0.55, P < 0.0001) for the same young subjects group was given in Figure 2, demonstrating consistency and reliability of vascular reactivity parameters at two visits.

Table 3. Within one-month repeatability scans and 18-month longitudinal mean percentage difference (2-1)/1 shown as Avg. % diff column, as well as two-time point (18-month follow-ups vs. 1st visits) mean comparison using paired t-test. MSE1 = mean square error of repeatability scans, MSE2 = mean square error of 18-month longitudinal scans, and fraction = MSE1/MSE2 SE=standard error. Significant longitudinal changes of test-retest samples (P<0.01) were highlighted in bold.

Parameter	Repeatability scans			Longitudinal data		
	MSE1	MSE2	Fraction	Avg. % diff	SE	P-value
Washout time (s)	0.05	1.04	0.05	6.5	1.2	0.81
Upslope (%/s)	0.13	0.99	0.13	-6.3	5.58	0.07
Overshoot (OS) (%)	0.22	0.72	0.31	-27.1	5.61	***0.003***
Pulse Ratio (PR)	0.02	0.16	0.11	5.1	3.50	***< 0.0001***
Forward flow time (T_{FF}, s)	0.16	0.32	0.48	2.6	5.81	0.53
Hyperemic index (HI)	0.17	0.29	0.60	-35.7	5.53	***< 0.0001***
Aortic PWV (aPWV, m/s)	0.09	0.16	0.57	-4.8	4.53	0.21
Thoraco-abdomin. PWV, daPWV	0.13	0.29	0.44	5.4	4.57	0.75
Iliofemoral PWV (ifPWV)	0.04	0.25	0.16	15.6	4.19	***0.0008***

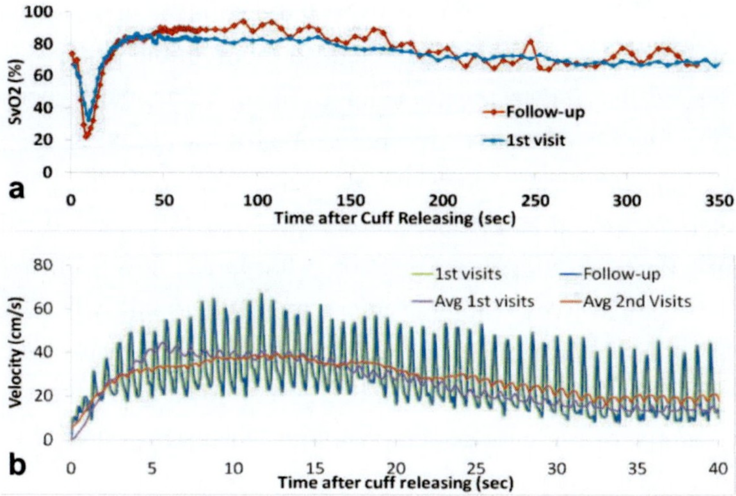

Figure 1. Demonstration of oximetry (a) and velocimetry (b) time curves at 1st and 2nd visits for the same non-smoking subject.

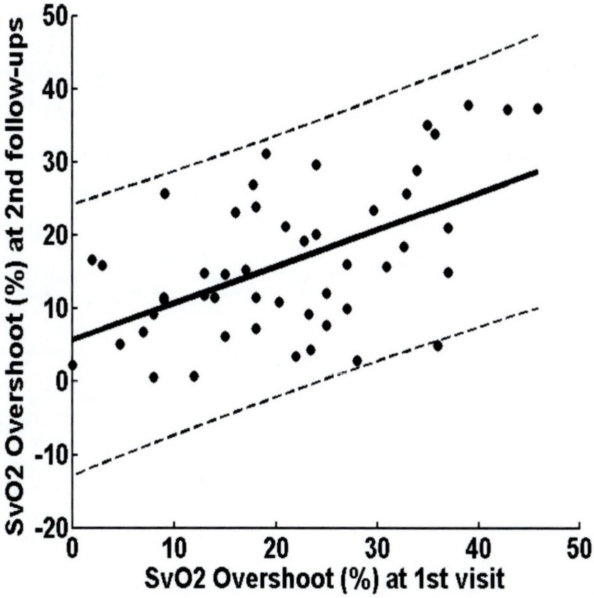

Figure 2. Significant correlation of SvO_2 overshoot between initial and follow-up visits ($r = 0.55$, $P < 0.0001$) indicated reliability of vascular reactivity parameters at two visits for the young subjects group.

3.2. Two-Way ANOVA Analysis and Two-sample *t*-Test

Table 4. Two-way ANOVA indicated that there was no significant interaction between smoking and age (P = 0.09-0.78) for all parameters evaluated at follow-ups

MRI Parameter	% Percentage Change = (group2-group1)/group1			t-test at 2nd visit P-value			
	YNS vs. ONS	YNS vs. YS	ONS vs. OS	Age & Smoking Interaction	YNS vs. ONS	YNS vs. YS	ONS vs. OS
Washout	30.48	-6.94	63.11	***0.26***	0.1841	0.2701	0.2279
Upslope	-15.87	-12.62	-25.09	***0.09***	0.0333	0.2539	0.0096
Overshoot	-26.64	-24.56	-7.95	***0.11***	0.0286	0.1229	0.6258
Pulse Ratio	18.27	13.99	-1.82	***0.31***	0.0009	0.0288	0.7306
T_{ff}	-10.75	-14.48	-1.18	***0.68***	0.2603	0.1804	0.9212
HI	-26.81	10.70	9.78	***0.26***	0.0114	0.4665	0.5214
aPWV	14.08	-1.60	8.16	***0.38***	0.0635	0.8675	0.3388
PWV-DA	34.04	19.58	5.00	***0.54***	<0.0001	0.1391	0.3497
PWV-IF	28.60	18.73	7.14	***0.26***	<0.0001	0.0271	0.2641
tPWV	26.88	11.70	4.40	***0.09***	<0.0001	0.0069	0.2260

At 2nd visit, similar to 1st visit, both aging and smoking effects were observed (P < 0.05), including decreased upslope in elderly group comparing to young group at non-smoker group (YNS vs. ONS, P = 0.03, percentage change = -15.9, purple color); and smoker group (ONS vs. OS, P = 0.03, percentage change = -25.1, red color). Other changes were decreased overshoot comparing YNS vs. ONS (P = 0.03, percentage change = -26.6), and increased pulse ratio comparing YNS vs. ONS (P = 0.0009, percentage change = -18.3) as well as comparing YNS vs. YS (P = 0.03, percentage change = -13.4). Hyperemia index (HI) was reduced comparing YNS vs. ONS (P = 0.01, percentage change = -26.8). Higher PWV at thoracoabdominal and iliofemoral sections as well as total PWV including aortic PWV comparing ONS vs. YNS (P < 0.0001), and comparing YNS vs. YS (P < 0.05) were found at 2nd visit as well.

Two-way ANOVA indicated that there was no significant interaction between smoking and age (P = 0.09-0.78) for all parameters evaluated at 2nd follow-up visits (Table 4). At 2nd visit, similar to 1st visit, both aging and smoking effects were observed (P < 0.05) with post-hoc two-sample t-test. For instance, most significant aging effects (about 27 years difference between old and young sub-groups) were found to the PWVs and pulse ratio (P<0.001).

3.3. One-way ANOVA Analysis at 2nd Visit Time

Table 5. Significant longitudinal effects by comparing 2nd visit to 1st visit were observed at follow-up times with 1-sample paired t-test

MRI Parameter	% Percentage Change btw visits = $(2^{nd}-1^{st})/1^{st}$ visit					Paired t-test (vs. 1st visit)				
	All	YNS N=39	YS N=14	ONS N=30	OS N=30	113 All Subjects	YNS N=39	YS N=14	ONS N=30	OS N=30
Washout	15.39	-7.76	-21.45	21.39	49.54	0.219	0.058	0.053	0.364	0.196
Upslope	-6.90	-16.36	-6.49	-0.74	-1.32	0.054	0.011	0.584	0.753	0.718
Overshoot	-11.91	-22.00	-18.82	-14.74	13.43	0.052	0.001	0.822	0.349	0.352
Pulse Ratio	2.31	-2.62	13.14	2.75	1.69	0.739	0.599	0.616	0.599	0.824
T_{ff}	-2.29	-2.67	-2.80	-8.93	0.67	0.644	0.929	0.797	0.713	0.683
HI	-42.69	-44.11	-22.52	-48.18	-48.16	<0.001	0.001	0.636	<0.001	0.038
aPWV	-9.87	-9.62	-15.48	-12.39	-6.02	0.005	0.112	0.012	0.045	0.775
PWV-DA	0.74	4.27	17.47	-1.06	-8.69	0.967	0.256	0.398	0.920	0.199
PWV-IF	11.73	6.45	13.90	11.89	17.11	<0.001	0.207	0.073	0.066	0.001
tPWV	4.67	2.63	8.35	4.88	4.15	0.113	0.481	0.142	0.350	0.602

Purple color indicates significant longitudinal effects in non-smoking groups and all subjects ($P < 0.05$).

Red color highlights significant longitudinal worsening ($P < 0.05$) in smokers (YS and OS) at follow-up times compared to their 1st visits.

Upslope, overshoot and HI were lower in YNS at 2nd visit compared to 1st visit. Shorter washout time, lower aortic PWV in YS but lower HI and higher iliofemoral PWV at OS groups comparing 2nd to 1st visits ($P < 0.05$).

Detailed significant between-group differences included: decreased upslope in elderly group comparing to young group at non-smoker group (YNS vs. ONS, P = 0.03, percentage change = -15.9); and smoker group (ONS vs. OS, P = 0.03, percentage change = -25.1).

Other changes include decreased overshoot comparing YNS vs. ONS (P = 0.03, percentage change = -26.6), and increased pulse ratio comparing YNS vs. ONS (P = 0.0009, percentage change = -18.3) as well as comparing YNS vs. YS (P = 0.03, percentage change = -13.4). Hyperemia index (HI) was reduced comparing YNS vs. ONS (P = 0.01, percentage change = -26.8). Higher PWV at thoracoabdominal and iliofemoral sections and total PWV including aortic PWV comparing ONS vs. YNS (P < 0.0001), as well as comparing YNS vs. YS (P < 0.05) were found at 2nd visit as well.

Significant longitudinal effects by comparing MRI parameters measured at 2nd visit to 1st visit were observed at non-smoking groups and all subjects (P < 0.05) with paired t-test (Table 5, purple color). And significant longitudinal worsening (P < 0.05) in smokers (YS and OS) at follow-up times was found as well compared to their 1st visit. Upslope, overshoot and HI were lower in YNS at 2nd visit compared to 1st visit. Shorter washout time, lower aortic PWV in YS, but lower HI and higher iliofemoral PWV in OS and ONS sub-groups were found at 2nd visit compared to baseline. Consistent with 1st visit, smokers and older subjects showed reduced vascular reactivity with lower arterial velocimetry and venous oximetry; as well as higher arterial stiffness measured with PWV at 18-month follow-ups. Representative examples of longitudinal changes of MRI parameters were illustrated, including decreased overshoot (Figure 3) and increased iliofemoral PWV (Figure 4) at 18-month follow-up in comparison to 1st visit in each sub-group and all subjects (P < 0.05). Similar to baseline findings, aging and smoking effects of overshoot (OS) and iliofemoral PWV were observed between sub-groups at 2nd visit (Table 4, Figure 3 and 4).

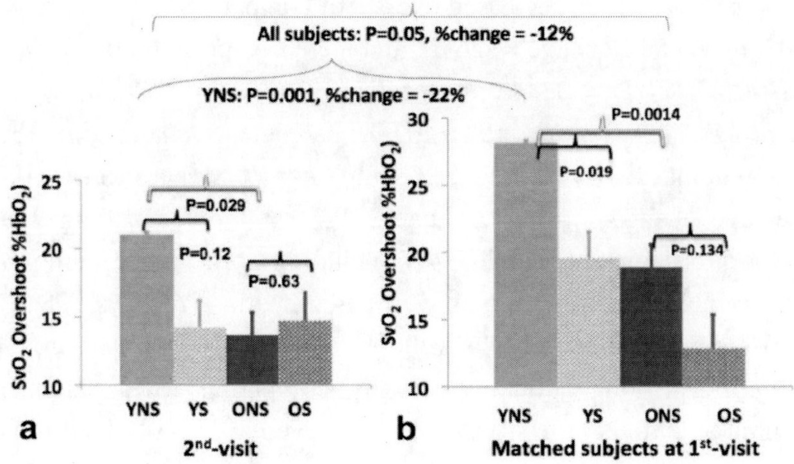

Figure 3. Paired t-test for the same MRI parameter between two visits across all subjects presented significant longitudinal worsening in several parameters including reduced SvO_2 overshoot (P = 0.05, percent change = -12%) for all subjects at 2nd visits (a), and most significant with P = 0.001 for young non-smokers sub-group (percent change = -22%). Aging effects were found at both visits, with more significant in the sub-group comparisons at 1st visit (b), and significant smoking effects of SvO_2 were only observed at 1st visit (b) comparing YS vs. YNS, possibly due to the less number of follow-up young sub-group subjects.

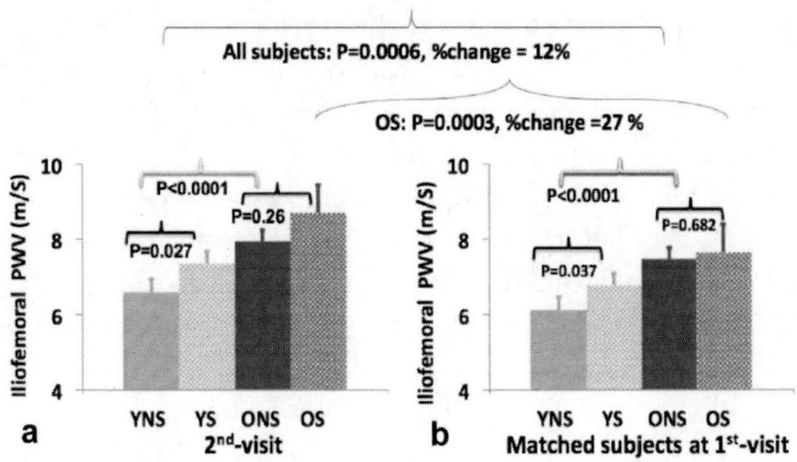

Figure 4. Paired t-test across all subjects showed significant longitudinal worsening in iliofemoral PWV (ifPWV, P = 0.0006, percent change = 12%) for all subjects, and especially in the old smokers group (P = 0.0003, percent change = 27%) at 2nd visits (a). Both aging and smoking effects between two sub-group comparisons were demonstrated for ifPWV at two visits, with significant differences between YNS and ONS (P < 0.0001) for two visits based on two-sample t-test, and significant differences between YNS vs. YS with P = 0.027 and P = 0.037 for 2nd visit (a) and 1st visit (b) respectively.

3.4. Correlation and Causality Analyses

Correlational analysis between 1st and 2nd visits showed significant influence of the small venous reactivity parameters (i.e., washout, upslope and overshoot) at 1st visit on the arterial stiffness parameters at follow-up visit (e.g., aortic arch, thoracoabdominal and iliofemoral PWVs) ($r > 0.29$, $P < 0.05$) (Table 6). Hyperemia index (HI) at 1st visit also correlated significantly with all the oximetry parameters at 2nd visits. Consistently, arterial stiffness parameters of the two visits correlated strongly with each other including aortic arch, thoracoabdominal and iliofemoral PWVs. Cross-vascular territories correlations of MRI parameters between two visits were found between upslope and OS at 1st and PWVs at 2nd visits. Similar correlations of inter-parameter correlations were observed of MRI measures involving the entire cohort at both visits.

Consistent with the baseline findings, significant correlations between MRI parameters and cardiovascular risk factors were found ($|r| > 0.2$,$P < 0.05$) at longitudinal follow-ups. Especially, significant correlations exist between systolic blood pressure (SBP) and upslope ($r = 0.37$, $P = 0.001$), C-reactive protein (CRP) and upslope ($r = 0.31$, $P = 0.005$), thoracoabdominal PWV and BMI ($r = -0.31$, $P = 0.0006$). Significant correlations were present between MRI hyperemic forward time (T_{ff}) parameter and all cardiovascular factors studied; for instance, between T_{ff} and SBP ($r = -0.36$, $P = 0.002$) as well as between T_{ff} and low-density lipoprotein cholesterol ($r = -0.27$, $P = 0.005$). And finally smoking severity (in pack years) was associated significantly with several MRI parameters including washout time ($r = 0.41$, $P = 0.008$), upslope ($r = -0.59$, $P < 0.0001$), overshoot ($r = -0.35$, $P = 0.03$), iliofemoral PWV ($r = 0.33$, $P = 0.04$) and total PWV ($r = 0.35$, $P = 0.03$) at 2nd visit.

Table 6. Micro- and macro- vasculature correlations between 1st visit (first column in yellow color) and 2nd visit (first column in green color and marked as metrics ending with "2"), as well as cross-correlations among parameters at 2nd visit

Correlation	Washout 2	Upslope 2	OS 2	Puls Ratio 2	TFF 2	HI 2	aPWV 2	PWV-DA 2	PWV-IF 2	tPWV 2
Washout	0.170	-0.242	-0.247	0.145	-0.166	-0.252	0.099	0.168	0.020	0.160
Upslope	-0.195	0.453	0.315	-0.265	0.198	0.073	-0.109	-0.332	-0.315	-0.434
OS	-0.274	0.330	0.401	-0.208	0.199	0.147	0.054	-0.357	-0.230	-0.325
Puls Ratio	0.123	0.027	-0.016	0.255	0.088	0.166	-0.037	0.278	0.170	0.242
TFF	-0.225	0.027	0.055	-0.044	0.373	0.232	0.008	-0.119	0.092	-0.080
HI	-0.121	0.252	0.179	-0.208	0.045	0.202	0.155	-0.067	0.052	0.024
aPWV	-0.111	-0.127	-0.091	-0.011	0.056	-0.012	0.207	0.236	0.132	0.184
PWV-DA	0.130	-0.202	-0.132	0.271	-0.061	-0.127	0.311	0.405	0.324	0.497
PWV-IF	0.002	-0.055	-0.021	0.226	0.119	-0.081	0.137	0.291	0.381	0.393
tPWV	0.065	-0.199	-0.096	0.237	0.033	-0.122	0.228	0.379	0.449	0.511
Washout 2	1.000	-0.045	-0.010	0.413	0.003	-0.107	0.067	0.355	0.277	0.262
Upslope 2	-0.045	1.000	0.548	-0.125	0.321	0.311	-0.006	-0.219	-0.162	-0.273
OS 2	-0.010	0.548	1.000	-0.147	0.231	0.190	0.004	-0.253	-0.147	-0.297
Puls Ratio 2	0.413	-0.125	-0.147	1.000	0.199	0.041	0.112	0.386	0.313	0.375
TFF 2	0.003	0.321	0.231	0.199	1.000	0.289	0.041	-0.093	0.165	-0.023
HI 2	-0.107	0.311	0.190	0.041	0.289	1.000	0.083	-0.041	-0.064	-0.107
aPWV 2	0.067	-0.006	0.004	0.112	0.041	0.083	1.000	0.157	0.141	0.386
PWV-DA 2	0.355	-0.219	-0.253	0.386	-0.093	-0.041	0.157	1.000	0.324	0.628
PWV-IF 2	0.277	-0.162	-0.147	0.313	0.165	-0.064	0.141	0.324	1.000	0.766
tPWV 2	0.262	-0.273	-0.297	0.375	-0.023	-0.107	0.386	0.628	0.766	1.000

- Green ($P<0.05$) and yellcw ($P<0.001$) numbers indicate significant correlations between each MRI parameter at 1st and 2nd visits.
- Blue ($P<0.05$) and light cyan ($P<0.001$) numbers indicate significant correlations between two MRI parameters within 2nd visits.

Significant correlations between each MRI parameter at 1st and 2nd visits were observed using causality analysis (upper-top section of the table, with green presents significance level of $P < 0.05$ and yellow for $P < 0.001$). Microvascular (i.e., small venous side) reactivity parameter including oximetry parameters (washout, upslope and overshoot-OS) at 1st visit had significant associations with almost all the vascular reactivity parameters at follow-up visits. Hyperemia index (HI) at 1st visit also correlated significantly with the oximetry parameters at 2nd visits. Consistently, arterial stiffness parameters of the 1st and 2nd visits correlated strongly with each other (aortic arch, thoracoabdominal, iliofemoral and total PWVs). Cross-vascular territories at two visits were found between oximetry including OS and upslope at 1st visit and PWVs at 2nd visit.

Regarding the causality correlations between cardiovascular risk factors, including total cholesterol, LDL, HDL, Triglycerides (TG), CRP, BMI, BP, and MRI metrics including microvascular parameters such as upslope and OS, as well as total PWV, significant correlations were found between cardiovascular risk factors at 1st visit and MRI parameters at 2nd visit follow-ups ($r > 0.19$, $P < 0.05$). Blood pressure and smoking pack years at 1st visit correlated significantly with most of MRI parameters at 18-month follow-ups. For instance, significant correlations were found between SBP at 1st visit and upslope at 2nd visit ($r = -0.36$, $P = 0.0001$), between SBP and tPWV ($r = 0.34$, $P = 0.0002$); as well as between pack years and tPWV ($r = 0.31$, $P = 0.001$).

4. Discussions and Conclusion

Our results confirmed that there were consistent EDF differences measured with MRI between smoker and non-smokers; and deterioration of EDF over 18 months period of follow-ups. Specifically, aging and smoking effects were found with multiple MRI VR assessments. For instance, decreased upslope and hyperemia index in elderly group comparing to young group at non-smoker group (YNS vs. ONS); and smoker group (YS vs. OS) at 2nd follow-up visit. Accompanying the micro-vascular VR changes, higher PWV at thoracoabdominal and iliofemoral sections as well as total PWV including aortic PWV comparing ONS to YNS were found as well ($P < 0.0001$). Microvascular oximetry parameters (washout, upslope and OS) at 1st visit correlated significantly with almost all the vascular reactivity parameters at 2nd visit, suggesting microvascular metrics might be a driven factor for the micro- and macro- vascular circulation characteristics sequentially.

Significant longitudinal worsening ($P < 0.05$) of EDF parameters in smokers at follow-up times was observed compared to their initial visit.

Upslope, overshoot, and HI were lower in YNS at 2nd visit compared to baseline. Shorter washout time, lower aortic PWV in YS but lower HI and higher iliofemoral PWV were found in OS groups 2nd visit. All longitudinal results indicated consistent age and smoking effects occur at a short 18-month time interval. Our results are in line with the previous brain study based on PET [^{15}-O]H_2O longitudinal data showing short-interval decreases in majority of brain regions including frontal, temporal and posterior cingulate cortices at 3.8 year interval using linear mixed effects model (Zhou et al. 2017). Sub-group comparison showed forward flow time (T_{ff}), hyperemic index (HI) and aortic arch PWV were worsening at follow-ups in smokers than non-smokers ($P < 0.05$). The main target toward assessment of micro-vascular reactivity and endothelial function was the femora popliteal circulation, given that atherosclerotic disease is far more prevalent in the lower than in upper extremities (Hickson et al. 2010; Langham et al. 2015). PWVs, especially iliofemoral PWV, were consistently higher in ONS group compared to YNS at both visits, suggesting possible atherosclerosis accumulation overtime with aging and smoking effects.

We also found significant correlations between multi-segmental PWVs, as well as between PWV and blood oxygenation metrics, further validating the robustness of our methods. An interesting observation is the association between the microvascular reactivity parameter derived from hyperemia (i.e., venous oxygen saturation overshoot and arterial velocity pulse ratio during hyperemia) and the multi-territorial macrovascular stiffness (i.e., thoracoabdominal PWV). Since both the pulse ratio and thoracoabdominal PWV reflected arterial wave propagation rate, these two parameters were significantly higher in older non-smokers compared to young healthy subjects. The correlations of microvascular and macrovascular parameters might suggest the co-occurrence of these two arterial vascular characteristics with both demonstrating compliance reduction at age (Talukder et al. 2011). However, in smokers, disassociation of these two vascular systems was found.

Both baseline and follow-up findings of the significant correlations among MRI parameters (e.g., PWV and T_{ff} and smoking severity suggest strong effects of smoking on MRI vascular reactivity parameters, especially arterial stiffness and speed. Our results were consistent with recent findings (Ijzerman et al. 2003; Doonan et al., 2010). And in line with previous imaging results, other cardiovascular disease factor parameters such as BMI, CRP, and cholesterol levels also showed significant smoking and aging effects (Langham et al. 2015; Mitchell et al. 2005). Furthermore, these biomarkers were significantly correlated with MRI parameters at both visits, indicating the microvascular compliance during hyperemia (i.e., oximetry and velocimetry) and macroscopic-level systematic mechanics (i.e., PWV) at different anatomical locations measured with MRI were both affected by the cardiovascular risk factors. Significant correlations between cardiovascular factors at initial visit and MRI parameters at 18-month follow-ups also implied that these risk factors (e.g., SBP and smoking pack years) could also be the causes of EDF including arterial stiffness measured with MRI with age and in smokers.

Our current results were mainly based on quantitative functional MRI data. As there are multiple causes that might lead to changes of the MRI vascular parameters, incorporating high-resolution structural and vessel wall imaging might help localize the underlying pathophysiological burdens (Hayes 2012; Kaul and Douglas 2009). Currently the number of participants in each sub-group is relatively small, and further collections of complete cardiovascular and metabolism data (especially smokers and other diseases including diabetes and obesity) with established and innovative MRI methods to corroborate current results are expected in the near future.

In conclusion, the vascular reactivity parameters in this study demonstrated significantly worsening of microvascular circulation and arterial stiffness with age and in smokers at 18-month follow-ups. These alterations are more likely to be resulted from atherosclerosis and cardiovascular risk increments over time in especially smokers and elderly people.

REFERENCES

[1] Ambrose JA, Barua RS. The pathophysiology of cigarette smoking and cardiovascular disease: an update. *J Am Coll Cardiol.* 2004;43:1731–7.

[2] Bernstein MA, King KF, Zhou ZJ. *Handbook of MRI pulse sequences.* Burlington, MA: Elsevier Academic Press; 2004. p. 669–71.

[3] Celermajer DS, Sorensen KE, Bull C, Robinson J, Deanfield JE. Endothelium- dependent dilation in the systemic arteries of asymptomatic subjects relates to coronary risk factors and their interaction. *J Am Coll Cardiol.* 1994;24:1468–74.

[4] Celermajer DS, Sorensen KE, Georgakopoulos D, Bull C, Thomas O, Robinson J, et al. Cigarette smoking is associated with dose-related and potentially reversible impairment of endothelium-dependent dilation in healthy young adults. *Circulation.* 1993;88:2149–55.

[5] Church DF, Pryor WA. Free-radical chemistry of cigarette smoke and its toxicological implications. *Environ Health Perspect.* 1985;64:111–26.

[6] Cooke JP, Dzau VJ. Nitric oxide synthase: role in the genesis of vascular disease. *Annu Rev Med.* 1997;48:489–509.

[7] Corretti MC, Anderson TJ, Benjamin EJ, Celermajer D, Charbonneau F, Creager MA, et al. Guidelines for the ultrasound assessment of endothelial- dependent flow-mediated vasodilation of the brachial artery: a report of the International Brachial Artery Reactivity Task Force. *J Am Coll Cardiol.* 2002;39:257–65.

[8] Davignon J, Ganz P. Role of endothelial dysfunction in atherosclerosis. *Circulation*. 2004;109:27–32.

[9] Doonan RJ, Hausvater A, Scallan C, Mikhailidis DP, Pilote L, Daskalopoulou SS. The effect of smoking on arterial stiffness. *Hypertens Res*. 2010;33:398–410.

[10] Fernandez-Seara MA, Techawiboonwong A, Detre JA, Wehrli FW. MR susceptometry for measuring global brain oxygen extraction. *Magn Reson Med*. 2006;55:967–73.

[11] Hallden S, Sjogren M, Hedblad B, Engstrom G, Narkiewicz K, Hoffmann M, et al. Smoking and obesity associated BDNF gene variance predicts total and cardiovascular mortality in smokers. *Heart*. 2013;99:949–53.

[12] Hamburg NM, Palmisano J, Larson MG, Sullivan LM, Lehman BT, Vasan RS, et al. Relation of brachial and digital measures of vascular function in the community: The Framingham heart study. *Hypertension*. 2011;57:390–6.

[13] Harris KF, Matthews KA. Interactions between autonomic nervous system activity and endothelial function: a model for the development of cardiovascular disease. *Psychosom Med*. 2004;66:153–64.

[14] Hickson SS, Butlin M, Graves M, Taviani V, Avolio AP, McEniery CM, et al. The relationship of age with regional aortic stiffness and diameter. *JACC Cardiovasc Imaging*. 2010;3:1247–55.

[15] Ijzerman RG, Serne EH, van Weissenbruch MM, de Jongh RT, Stehouwer CD. Cigarette smoking is associated with an acute impairment of microvascular function in humans. *Clin Sci* (Lond). 2003;104:247–52.

[16] Kaul P, Douglas PS. Atherosclerosis imaging: prognostically useful or merely more of what we know? *Circ Cardiovasc Imaging*. 2009;2:150–60.

[17] Kiowski W, Linder L, Stoschitzky K, Pfisterer M, Burckhardt D, Burkart F, et al. Diminished vascular response to inhibition of

endothelium-derived nitric oxide and enhanced vasoconstriction to exogenously administered endothelin-1 in clinically healthy smokers. *Circulation*. 1994;90:27–34.

[18] Langham MC, Magland JF, Floyd TF, Wehrli FW. Retrospective correction for induced magnetic field inhomogeneity in measurements of large-vessel hemoglobin oxygen saturation by MR susceptometry. *Magn Reson Med*. 2009;61:626–33.

[19] Langham MC, Floyd TF, Mohler 3rd ER, Magland JF, Wehrli FW. Evaluation of cuff-induced ischemia in the lower extremity by magnetic resonance oximetry. *J Am Coll Cardiol*. 2010;55:598–606.

[20] Langham MC, Li C, Wehrli FW. Non-triggered quantification of central and peripheral pulse-wave velocity. *J Cardiovasc Magn Reson*. 2011;13:81.

[21] Langham MC, Zhou Y, Chirico EN, Magland JF, Sehgal CM, Englund EK, Mohler III ER, Guo W, Wehrli FW, Effects of Age and Smoking on End othelial Function Assessed by Quantitative MRI and Ultrasound in the Peripheral and Central Vasculature", *Journal of Cardiovascular Magnetic Resnance*, 2015; 17(1):19, 201546.

[22] Laurent S, Cockcroft J, Van Bortel L, Boutouyrie P, Giannattasio C, Hayoz D, et al. Expert consensus document on arterial stiffness: methodological issues and clinical applications. *Eur Heart J*. 2006;27:2588–605.

[23] Mitchell GF, Vita JA, Larson MG, Parise H, Keyes MJ, Warner E, et al. Cross-sectional relations of peripheral microvascular function, cardiovascular disease risk factors, and aortic stiffness: the Framingham Heart Study. *Circulation*. 2005;112:3722–8.

[24] Pencina MJ, D'Agostino Sr RB, Larson MG, Massaro JM, Vasan RS. Predicting the 30-year risk of cardiovascular disease: the framingham heart study. *Circulation*. 2009;119:3078–84.

[25] Talukder MA, Johnson WM, Varadharaj S, Lian J, Kearns PN, El-Mahdy MA, et al. Chronic cigarette smoking causes hypertension,

increased oxidative stress, impaired NO bioavailability, endothelial dysfunction, and cardiac remodeling in mice. *Am J Physiol Heart Circ Physiol.* 2011;300:H388–96.

[26] WHO urges more countries to require large, graphic health warnings on tobacco packaging: the WHO report on the global tobacco epidemic, 2011 examines anti-tobacco mass-media campaigns. *Cent Eur J Public Health* 2011, 19:133, 151.http://www.ncbi.nlm.nih.gov/ pumed/ 22026286.

[27] Wiesmann F, Petersen SE, Leeson PM, Francis JM, Robson MD, Wang Q, et al. Global impairment of brachial, carotid, and aortic vascular function in young smokers: direct quantification by high-resolution magnetic resonance imaging. *J Am Coll Cardiol.* 2004;44:2056–64.

[28] Wilkinson IB, Fuchs SA, Jansen IM, Spratt JC, Murray GD, Cockcroft JR, et al. Reproducibility of pulse wave velocity and augmentation index measured by pulse wave analysis. *J Hypertens*. 1998;16:2079–84.

[29] Zhou Y, Rodgers ZB, and Kuo AH, Cerebrovascular Reactivity Measured with Arterial Spin Labeling and Blood Oxygen Level Dependent Techniques", *Magnetic Resonance Imaging*, 2015; 22(5):566-576.

[30] Zhou Y, Cerebral Blood Flow Mediated Rapid Vascular Reactivity Mapping and Effects of Age and Smoking", in *Horizons in Neuroscience Research*. Vol. 31, Chapter III, Nova Science Publishers, 2017.

[31] Zhou Y, *Functional Neuroimaging Methods and Frontiers*, Nova Science Publishers, 2018.

[32] Zhou Y, *Functional Neuroimaging with Multiple Modalities: Principles, Device and Applications*, Nova Science Publishers, 2016.

[33] Zhou Y, *Neuroimaging in Multiple Sclerosis*, Nova Science Publishers, 2017.

Chapter 4

Longitudinal Changes of Molecular Imaging and Correlations among PET/MRI Metrics

Abstract

Prior studies have shown that the hazard ratio increases linearly with the number of risk factors, including cerebrovascular disease, tau and amyloid burden. In this chapter, we will report longitudinal changes of molecular imaging tracers including tau, amyloid and [^{18}-F]Fluoro-2-deoxyglucose (FDG) quantifications from the ADNI cohort in addition to our previous baseline aging findings. Regarding MRI and PET imaging correlations, our aims are to compare the white matter (WM) lesion volume, amyloid burden, FDG glucose uptake in patients with early Alzheimer's disease (AD), mild cognitive impairment (MCI) and healthy controls. And the correlations among WM lesion volume with amyloid burden, FDG uptake as well as functional connectivity changes in MCI and early AD patients will be examined further. Longitudinal tau changes (0.1-1.5% yearly rate of increment) demonstrated a posterior to anterior occipito-temporal degradation pattern at different follow-up times in comparison to baseline. All longitudinal results indicated most significant progression of tau deposition was present in the Braak stage IV regions including temporal pole and middle temporal cortex. Decrement of tau deposition in the early transentorhinal region and fusiform at follow-ups could possibly due to the spreading effects from these earlier Braak stage regions (I & III) to relatively later stage regions such as temporal poles. Significant longitudinal changes of regional amyloid deposition demonstrated about 0.3-0.4% beta-amyloid increment at 24-month follow-up times in the temporal cortex, especially in the middle and inferior temporal sub-segments, compared to baseline. The whole brain cerebrum had about 0.1% increment including regions of bilateral parsorbitalis (about 0.45% biyearly rate) and right lateral occipital cortex (0.15% rate). As for FDG glucose metabolism, longitudinal data found significant reductions (most of $P \leq 0.0001$) of glucose metabolic rate at variable follow-up times in the regions of bilateral temporal, angular and posterior cortices. The rate of FDG metabolism decline varied slightly for different regions, with about -1.6% every year decline of glucose metabolic rate for the posterior cingulum and -1.3% yearly for left temporal cortex, -1.9% yearly for bilateral angular region. Based on ADNI2 cohort data, there is no longitudinal change of global white matter hyperintensity at 3 to 24 months time interval compared to baseline ($P > 0.05$). Regarding the correlations between different imaging parameters, aside from significant associations between tau and other imaging metrics, significant correlation was found between white matter lesion load (WMLL) and amyloid load averaged over the whole cerebral cortex in all three groups combining controls, MCI and AD (Pearson $r = 0.46$, $P = 0.015$; Spearman rank $r = 0.46$, $P = 0.013$). A negative correlation between FDG uptake and amyloid load was noted in all three groups ($r = -0.57$, $P = 0.0006$).

Taken together, there are variable degrees of longitudinal changes regarding to higher tau deposition, amyloid accumulation and FDG hypometabolism with age. The concurrence of WM hyperintensity, gray matter atrophy, structural disconnectivity and functional hyper-perfusion s well as higher tau, amyloid and lower FDG in entorhinal, hippocampal and other temporal regions suggested detectable pathological, structural and functional brain changes at both molecular and macroscopic levels, at even early stages of dementia including MCI patients.

1. INTRODUCTION

The pathological hallmarks of early Alzheimer's disease (AD) are amyloid plaques and mis-folded tau tangles (Braak and Braak 1991). We have recently investigated multiple MRI and conventional PET imaging biomarkers (e.g., amyloid and glucose metabolism) for differentiating early AD from normal controls and mild cognitive impairment (MCI) patients. These multiple metrics include structural and functional connectivity based on MRI (fcMRI), functional activity, small-worldness analysis with MRI cortical thickness to better identify several stages of early dementia, white matter lesion load (a marker for cerebrovascular risk), as well as PET amyloid and tau load for better understanding and defining the underlying neuropathological changes of brain circuits and association with phenotypic data (Zhou et al. 2008; Zhou et al. 2015; Zhou 2016). The between-modality interactions including human brain structural and functional networks undergo robust changes in normal aging and preclinical stages of AD, suggesting that neuroimaging metrics and combination from various networks in different scales might be useful to monitor brain changes (Zhou et al. 2015). A recent study found partial interaction between longitudinal perfusion and glucose metabolism maps, with overlaps between perfusion and tau only in the temporal areas (Leuzy et al. 2018). Primary age-related taupathy (PART) and staging of tau as well as in vivo associations between tau and MRI metrics had recently been reported (Zhou et al. 2017a). Due to the relatively new development of the tau tracer, longitudinal studies of multiple imaging metrics need to be further quantified and confirmed.

As illustrated in the hypothetical model, compared to other PET tracers including beta- amyloid (Aβ), [^{18}-F] Fluoro-2-deoxyglucose (FDG) and MRI structural/functional biomarkers, the intracellular tau deposition had been assumed to be particularly sensitive in the prodromal stage, especially the pre-clinical and MCI stages (Ariza et al. 2015; Barret et al. 2016). The difficulties of labeling intracellular tau neurofibrillary tangle (NFT) deposition include requirement of high specificity of the tracer over the other five tau isoforms and enough abundance of the binding of the tracer to the intracellular tau (Brendel et al. 2016; Brier et al. 2016). The tracer molecular size needs to be small enough and designed to be lipophilic to cross the blood brain barrier (BBB) and cell membrane, to bind to the paired-helical filaments (PHF)-tau selectively (Chiotis et al. 2016). It has been recently reported that PET [^{18}-F]AV-1451 tracer binds tau avidly to 3R+4R tau in the form of NFT, and more specifically to AD type neurodegenerative disease than other types, especially in the early stages of dementia (Lowe et al. 2016). Most other tauopathies are characterized by the presence of both neuronal and glial tau pathologies (Kahlson and Colodner, 2015). With the development of tracer labeling and imaging techniques, over the past two decades, there are quite a few recent studies reported that successfully imaged tau depositions, especially the intracellular PHF which are insoluble fibers composed of hyper-phosphorylated tau, in MCI and Alzheimer's disease (AD); and correlated with several cognitive tests (Clavaguera et al. 2010; Holmes et al. 2016). However, due to recent availability of the PET tracer, there are very limited numbers of participants studied and most of them were relatively elderly (Jack et al. 2010; Jack et al. 2013; Jack et al. 2016; Kahlson et al. 2015).

Another potential risk factor associated with aging is microvascular disease (Zhou et al. 2015). White matter (WM) lesion, detected as WM hyperintensities (WMH) on MRI T2-weighted images, may represent microvascular ischemic and/or demyelinating changes (Chui, 2006) and in which case they can be considered a marker for cerebrovascular disease (CVD) (Debette and Markus, 2010; Wardlaw et al. 2013). In the elderly population, WM lesions are believed to be potential risk factors for memory and cognitive impairment (Geppert et al. 2007). WMH have been found to be associated with an increased incidence of dementia (Brickman et al. 2012), as well as the development of WM microstructural changes in the presymptomatic stage of disease (Ryan et al. 2011). Utilizing diffusion tensor imaging (DTI), age-related WM degeneration (i.e., fractional anisotropy and diffusivity) has been identified, particularly in the prefrontal cortex and splenium of corpus callosum (Salat et al. 2005). DTI tractography of the posterior cingulate and hippocampal WM regions in MCI and early AD demonstrate reduced fiber tract numbers as well, consistent with reduced functional connectivity noted on fMRI (Zhou et al. 2008). A negative correlation between, WMH lesions and fMRI blood oxygen-level dependent (BOLD) signal in elderly individuals performing episodic memory or finger tapping tasks has been reported in the prefrontal and parietal regions (Nordahl et al. 2006; Patel et al. 2012). Greater WMH lesion burden were also found in elderly individuals with microbleeds based on MRI T2* gradient echo and susceptibility weighted images, suggesting a possible microhemorrhage contribution to WMH in aging (Whitwell et al. 2013). These results suggest that there are WM micro-structural and cerebrovascular disruptions in both elderly and demented subjects. However, the threshold separating WM lesion burden in the normal elderly population and dementia/AD patients has yet to be determined.

A significant relationship between the composite AD pathological score at autopsy and white matter disease score from T2-weighted MRI images was found among a cohort of elderly subjects (Moghekar et al. 2012). Amyloid plaque distribution patterns have been found to co-localize with resting state (RS)-fMRI core hub regions such as the default mode network (DMN), even before the clinical onset of disease (Buckner et al. 2005). Furthermore, hypometabolism based on [^{18}F]-FDG PET measuring metabolic rate of glucose (CMRglu), which is considered a marker of neuronal dysfunction has been shown to be a prominent feature in early AD, particularly in the posterior parietal and cingulate regions (Silverman et al. 2001). Although the extracellular amyloid deposition is not directly correlated with detectable vascular injury (i.e., cerebral amyloid angiopathy, CAA) (Takada et al. 2009), its association with white matter damage and resting-state (RS)-fMRI changes including default mode network (DMN) functional connectivity (Zhou et al. 2015) and functional activity measured with fractional amplitude at low-frequency fluctuation (fALFF) at different stages of dementia, needs to be further examined.

Prior studies have shown that the hazard ratio increases linearly with the number of risk factors, including cerebrovascular disease and amyloid burden (Reed et al. 2012). Significant correlations among multiple imaging metrics are expected, and the integration points to the possibility of earlier diagnosis and prevention. In addition to our previous baseline findings (Zhou et al. 2015; Zhou et al. 2017b), we will report the longitudinal changes over 1-6 years follow-up times of molecular imaging tracers including tau, amyloid, FDG as well as WMH quantifications from the Alzheimer's Disease Neuroimaging Initiative (ADNI) cohort in this chapter. And the correlations among WM lesion volume with amyloid burden, tau and FDG uptake as well as functional connectivity changes in MCI and early AD patients will be examined further.

2. Method

Data used in the preparation of this article were obtained from the Alzheimer's Disease Neuroimaging Initiative (ADNI) database (adni.loni.usc.edu). The ADNI was launched in 2003 as a public-private partnership, led by Principal Investigator Michael W. Weiner, MD. The primary goal of ADNI has been to test whether serial magnetic resonance imaging (MRI), positron emission tomography (PET), other biological markers, and clinical and neuropsychological assessment can be combined to measure the progression of MCI and early AD. Preprocessed study data of healthy elderly and early AD (mostly preclinical participants) including tau, amyloid, FDG and WMH were downloaded with permission and analyzed with in-house statistical tools for region of interest (ROI) quantification, longitudinal analysis and regional coherence computation.

3. Results

3.1. Tau Imaging

Longitudinal follow-up AV-[1451] tau imaging data analysis had been performed to the ADNI cohort for available participants. 87 participants had longitudinal data with following up times ranging from 10 months to 48 months (1 participant with 10 months follow-up, 65 participants with 12 months follow-up, 1 with 14 months, 18 for 24 months, 1 at 36 months and 1 at 48 months).

Significant longitudinal changes of regional tau standard uptake value ratio (SUVR) choosing cerebellum as reference were listed in Table 1 with $P < 0.05$ for different follow-up times. Table 1a listed longitudinal changes of tau for all participants with mean follow-up time of 15.4 months. Longitudinal tau changes at rate of about 0.1-1.5% yearly demonstrated a posterior to anterior and occipito-temporal degradation pattern at different follow-up times in comparison to baseline. Higher tau tangles in the lingual, cuneous and precuneous regions were observed at 12-month follow-ups (Table 1b). At 24-months follow-up time, higher tau tangles in the temporal cortex including bilateral temporal pole were found, with slightly less tau depositions in the entorhinal cortex, fusiform and inferior temporal regions compared to baseline (Table 1c). All longitudinal results indicated that most significant progression of tau deposition was present in the Braak stage IV regions including temporal pole and middle temporal cortex. Decrement of tau deposition in the early transentorhinal region and fusiform at follow-ups could possibly due to the spreading effects from these earlier Braak stage regions (I & III) to relatively later stage regions such as temporal poles.

In addition, similar to functional connectivity application, we found significant correlations between hippocampal tau and tau depositions in other brain regions ($r > 0.3$, $P < 0.0001$) across subjects. The highly significant correlations were presented mostly in cortical areas, excluding a few non-significant off-target sub-cortical regions such as caudate and pallidum. Similar correlations were found based on volumetry; for instance, most significance were found between volumes of hippocampus and entorhinal cortex/amydala ($r > 0.5$, $P < 0.00001$), but non-significant between volume of hippocampus and volumes of thalamus, choroid (CSF), brain stem and white matter. These results implicate that regional cortical coherence and data consistency were maintained using intracellular neuropathological burden quantifications.

Table 1a. Significant tau SUVR differences (P < 0.05) and percentage change (%) between longitudinal follow-up images (mean follow-up time = 15.2 months) and baseline for available 87 subjects showed a posteriorto anterior and occipito-temporal degradation pattern SUVR=standard uptake value ratio choosing cerebellum as reference region, LH=left hemisphere, RH=right hemisphere. Significant more accumulation of longitudinal cortical tau tangles in gray matter regions were highlighted in gray color (P<0.05)

ROI name	P-value	% Change
CC_CENTRAL_SUVR	0.0157	1.8205
CC_MID_ANTERIOR_SUVR	0.0466	-0.5824
CC_MID_POSTERIOR_SUVR	0.0009	0.1152
CSF_SUVR	0.0024	4.3541
CTX_LH_CUNEUS_SUVR	0.0246	1.8581
CTX_LH_ENTORHINAL_SUVR	0.0146	-2.184
CTX_LH_INFERIORTEMPORAL_SUVR	0.0358	-3.5174
CTX_LH_MIDDLETEMPORAL_SUVR	0.0419	0.0912
LEFT_CHOROID_PLEXUS_SUVR	0.0149	-0.1963
LEFT_LATERAL_VENTRICLE_SUVR	0.0003	4.6085
NON_WM_HYPOINTENSITIES_SUVR	0.0275	0.6373
RIGHT_CHOROID_PLEXUS_SUVR	0.0044	-2.8337
RIGHT_LATERAL_VENTRICLE_SUVR	0.0001	0.8655

Table 1b. Significant tau differences between baseline and 12-month follow-ups (P < 0.05, N = 65)

ROI names	P-value	% Change
CC_CENTRAL_SUVR	0.0242	1.3157
CC_MID_ANTERIOR_SUVR	0.041	-0.999
CC_MID_POSTERIOR_SUVR	0.0013	-0.0086
CC_POSTERIOR_SUVR	0.0135	-0.9459
CSF_SUVR	0.0059	3.5596
CTX_LH_CUNEUS_SUVR	0.002	0.97
CTX_LH_LINGUAL_SUVR	0.0113	0.5304
CTX_LH_PRECUNEUS_SUVR	0.0188	1.2849
CTX_RH_CUNEUS_SUVR	0.0043	-0.1985
CTX_RH_LINGUAL_SUVR	0.009	0.1831
CTX_RH_PERICALCARINE_SUVR	0.0072	-0.8466
CTX_RH_TRANSVERSETEMPORAL	0.0199	-0.398
LEFT_CAUDATE_SUVR	0.029	-0.2226
LEFT_CHOROID_PLEXUS_SUVR	0.0092	-0.6962
LEFT_LATERAL_VENTRICLE_SUVR	0.0001	2.489
LEFT_VENTRALDC_SUVR	0.0485	0.3634
RIGHT_CHOROID_PLEXUS_SUVR	0.0016	-1.3713
RIGHT_LATERAL_VENTRICLE	0.0004	0.1646

Table 1c. Significant tau differences between baseline and 24-month follow-ups (P < 0.05, N = 18)

ROI name	P-value	% Change
CTX_LH_ENTORHINAL_SUVR	0.0244	-1.9616
CTX_LH_FUSIFORM_SUVR	0.0242	-0.5967
CTX_LH_INFERIORTEMPORAL_SUVR	0.01	-3.9656
CTX_LH_TEMPORALPOLE_SUVR	0.0308	0.4622
CTX_RH_TEMPORALPOLE_SUVR	0.0085	1.3227
NON_WM_HYPOINTENSITIES_SUVR	0.0186	1.5386
RIGHT_LATERAL_VENTRICLE_SUVR	0.0293	2.4241

On the other hand, there is almost no overlap between tau deposition and microhemorrhage (MCH) detected with MRI gradient recalled echo (GRE)-T2* sequence. This is mainly due to the reason that MCH are presented mostly in deep gray matter in these preclinical participants.

3.2. Amyloid Imaging

Table 2a. Significant amyloid SUVR differences (P < 0.005) between baseline and follow-ups for available 1018 subjects (mean follow-up time = 24.4 months)
Significant more deposition of longitudinal cortical amyloid in gray matter regions were highlighted in gray color (P<0.05).

ROI name	P-value	% Change
TEMPORAL	0.0046	0.3114
SUMMARYSUVR_WHOLECEREBNORM	0.0036	0.1176
SUMMARYSUVR_COMPOSITE_REFNORM	0.0007	-0.2846
CTX_LH_BANKSSTS	0.0025	0.2913
CTX_LH_FUSIFORM	0.0042	0.0289
CTX_LH_INFERIORTEMPORAL	0.0012	0.158
CTX_LH_LATERALOCCIPITAL	0.0016	-0.0615
CTX_LH_LINGUAL	0.0043	-0.1263
CTX_LH_MIDDLETEMPORAL	0.0015	0.282
CTX_LH_PARSORBITALIS	0.0026	0.4152
CTX_LH_PERICALCARINE	0.0027	-0.0584
CTX_RH_INFERIORTEMPORAL	0.0038	0.4141
CTX_RH_LATERALOCCIPITAL	0.0048	0.1532
CTX_RH_MIDDLETEMPORAL	0.0032	0.391
CTX_RH_PARSORBITALIS	0.0036	0.5342
LEFT_CHOROID_PLEXUS	0.0013	4.8155
LEFT_LATERAL_VENTRICLE	0.001	8.5681
RIGHT_CHOROID_PLEXUS	0.0027	5.1857
RIGHT_LATERAL_VENTRICLE	0.0012	8.2716
WM_HYPOINTENSITIES	0.0012	4.8243

Significant longitudinal changes of regional amyloid SUVR deposition were listed in Table 2 (P < 0.005 and range of follow-up times is 12-70 months) for available 1018 subjects with mean follow-up time of 24.4 months (Table 2a). Longitudinal changes demonstrated about 0.3-0.4% beta-amyloid deposition increment at 24-month follow-up times in the temporal cortex, especially in the middle and inferior temporal sub-segments, compared to baseline (Table 2b).

Table 2b. Significant amyloid differences between baseline and 24-month follow-up (P < 0.005, N = 919)

ROI name	P-value	% Change
SUMMARYSUVR_COMPOSITE_REFNORM	0.0014	-0.2313
CTX_LH_BANKSSTS	0.0048	0.3524
CTX_LH_INFERIORTEMPORAL	0.0033	0.2984
CTX_LH_LATERALOCCIPITAL	0.002	-0.1372
CTX_LH_MIDDLETEMPORAL	0.0034	0.3738
CTX_RH_LATERALOCCIPITAL	0.0048	0.0416
LEFT_CHOROID_PLEXUS	0.0004	5.3592
LEFT_LATERAL_VENTRICLE	0.0002	9.5217
RIGHT_CHOROID_PLEXUS	0.0014	5.6875
RIGHT_LATERAL_VENTRICLE	0.0003	9.1874
WM_HYPOINTENSITIES	0.0002	5.4059

Table 2c. Significant amyloid differences between baseline and 12-month follow-up (P < 0.005, N = 55)

ROI name	P-value	% Change
CC_MID_ANTERIOR	0.0034	-4.3814
CC_MID_POSTERIOR	0.0023	-4.338
CSF	0.0018	-3.4764
CTX_LH_UNKNOWN	0.0027	-2.6438
LEFT_AMYGDALA	0.0026	-2.6792
LEFT_CAUDATE	0.0004	-4.699
LEFT_CHOROID_PLEXUS	0.0003	-4.8307
LEFT_HIPPOCAMPUS	0.004	-2.4174
LEFT_INF_LAT_VENT	0.0024	-3.0592
LEFT_LATERAL_VENTRICLE	0.0001	-7.0782
NON_WM_HYPOINTENSITIES	0.0002	-5.5453
RIGHT_CAUDATE	0.0001	-4.7497
RIGHT_CHOROID_PLEXUS	0.0018	-4.4723
RIGHT_LATERAL_VENTRICLE	0.0001	-6.7596
RIGHT_THALAMUS_PROPER	0.0032	-2.5715
WM_HYPOINTENSITIES	0.0014	-4.4385

3.3. FDG Imaging

Table 3. Significant FDG glucose hypo-metabolism SUVR (P < 0.005) at follow-up visits compared to baseline for available 2051 subjects (mean follow-up times = 14.7 months) using regional mean, median and mode metrics

Follow-up Time Points	6-months		12-months		24 months		Mean 14.7 months	
Region and Metric	P-value	% Change	P-value	% Change	P-value	% Change	P-value	% Change
Mean Left Angular	<0.0001	-0.9820	<0.0001	-2.0594	<0.0001	-2.8765	<0.0001	-2.0258
Mean Right Angular	<0.0001	-1.0111	<0.0001	-1.4309	<0.0001	-2.6359	<0.0001	-1.8822
Mean Posterior Cingulate	<0.0001	-1.2523	<0.0001	-1.7368	<0.0001	-3.2484	<0.0001	-2.2361
Mean Left Temporal	<0.0001	-0.9622	<0.0001	-2.0885	<0.0001	-2.6118	<0.0001	-1.8848
Mean Right Temporal	<0.0001	-0.8373	0.0001	-1.3008	<0.0001	-2.0323	<0.0001	-1.4937
Median Left Angular	<0.0001	-0.9703	<0.0001	-2.0764	<0.0001	-2.8627	<0.0001	-2.0161
Median Right Angular	<0.0001	-1.0165	<0.0001	-1.4371	<0.0001	-2.6722	<0.0001	-1.8981
Median Posterior Cingulate	<0.0001	-1.2543	<0.0001	-1.6976	<0.0001	-3.1554	<0.0001	-2.1966
Median Left Temporal	<0.0001	-0.9705	<0.0001	-2.0834	<0.0001	-2.5914	<0.0001	-1.8806
Median Right Temporal	<0.0001	-0.8578	0.0001	-1.3094	<0.0001	-2.0011	<0.0001	-1.4888
Mode Left Angular	0.0024	-0.6793	0.0002	-1.5269	<0.0001	-2.2209	<0.0001	-1.5612
Mode Right Angular	0.0482	-0.2616	0.0353	-0.8493	0.0001	-1.8189	<0.0001	-1.1867
Mode Posterior Cingulate	0.0001	-1.1608	0.0883	-0.5876	<0.0001	-3.7883	<0.0001	-2.1958
Mode Left Temporal	<0.0001	-0.8873	<0.0001	-2.0575	<0.0001	-2.4371	<0.0001	-1.7825
Mode Right Temporal	0.0010	-0.6163	0.0026	-1.0495	<0.0001	-1.9519	<0.0001	-1.3003

The whole brain cerebrum had about 0.12% increment including regions of bilateral parsorbitalis (about 0.45% biyearly or 0.23% yearly rate) and right lateral occipital cortex (0.15% rate) over 24 months.

Regional connectivity results indicated high coherence between hippocampal amyloid SUVR and other brain regions; most significant in cortical areas ($r>0.3$, $P<0.0001$) excluding the subcortical caudate and pallidum regions. Similar to tau images, cortical coherences of amyloid distribution across subjects were also maintained based on SUVR and volumetry.

As for FDG glucose metabolism, longitudinal data of 2051 follow-ups with mean 14.7 months showed significant reduction (most significance levels are $P \leq 0.0001$) of metabolic rate at variable follow-up times (6, 12 and 24 months) in the regions of bilateral temporal, angular and posterior cortices (Table 3). The rate of decline (regional average) varied slightly for different regions, with about -1.6% every year decline rate of mean glucose metabolism for the posterior cingulum and -1.3% yearly for left temporal cortex, -1.9% yearly for bilateral angular region. Similar hypometabolic degrees at follow-ups were observed using the median and mode metrics in these regions as well.

Regional connectivity results indicated high coherence between hippocampal FDG SUVR and other brain regions; most significant in cortical areas ($r > 0.3$, $P < 0.0001$) excluding the subcortical caudate and pallidum regions. Similar to tau imaging, cortical coherence was also maintained based on volumetry.

3.4. White Matter Lesion Load (WMLL)

WM lesions, indicated as WMH on the FLAIR images, were downloaded from ADNI and segmented semi-automatically (manual outlining with white matter intensity constraints) using FireVoxel software for each subject (Mikheev et al. 2008). The whole brain white matter lesion load (WMLL) was obtained as the volume (in units of milliliter, ml) of the hyper-intense (≥ mean+2.5 standard deviation) voxels in WM. Then the lesion map generated from the FLAIR images was co-registered to MPRAGE data of each subject and normalized to the Montreal Neurological Institute (MNI) 2mm standard space in FSL using a nonlinear warping algorithm. Finally, the lesion probability map (LPM) was generated by averaging the binarized normalized lesion maps within each group (Zhou et al. 2015).

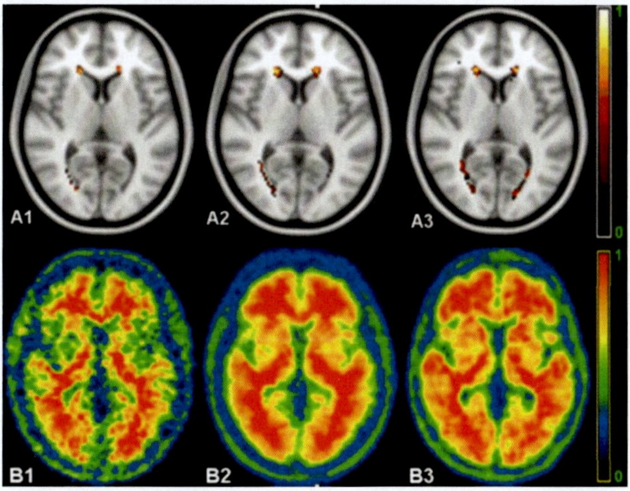

Source and color image: Adapted from Zhou Y, Yu F, Duong TQ, Alzheimer's Disease Neuroimaging Initiative (2015) White matter lesion load is associated with resting state functional MRI activity and amyloid PET but not FDG in mild cognitive impairment and early Alzheimer's disease patients. *J Magn Reson Imaging* 41:102-109. Used with permission.

Figure 1. A: Representative axial slice of lesion probability map (LPM) in each group based on MRI T2-FLAIR images showed a peri-ventricular WM lesion distribution. Compared to controls (A1), LPM in MCI (A2) and AD (A3) groups showed significantly increased WM lesions in especially the left periventricular WM around the occipital horn and frontal WM. B: Amyloid imaging using PET [^{18}F]-Florbetapir tracer in the normal control (B1), MCI (B2), and AD (B3) subjects showed increased amyloid deposition patterns in MCI patients in medial frontal and parietal regions; and increased uptake in almost the whole brain in AD patients. Amyloid deposition was averaged across subjects in each group after normalizing with the maximal value individually.

Based on the FLAIR images, a varying degree of peri-ventricular and frontal white matter lesions in AD and MCI patients as well as controls were identified (Figure 1a). However based on ADNI2 cohort data, no significant longitudinal change of WMLL is found at 3 to 24 months time interval compared to baseline ($P > 0.05$) despite the group differences between controls and MCI/early AD at baseline. Quantitative whole brain WMLL was significantly higher in patients with MCI (12.88 ± 7.47 ml) and AD (13.16 ± 5.12 ml) than controls (5.15 ± 2.41 ml) (Figure 2), both with $P < 0.005$.

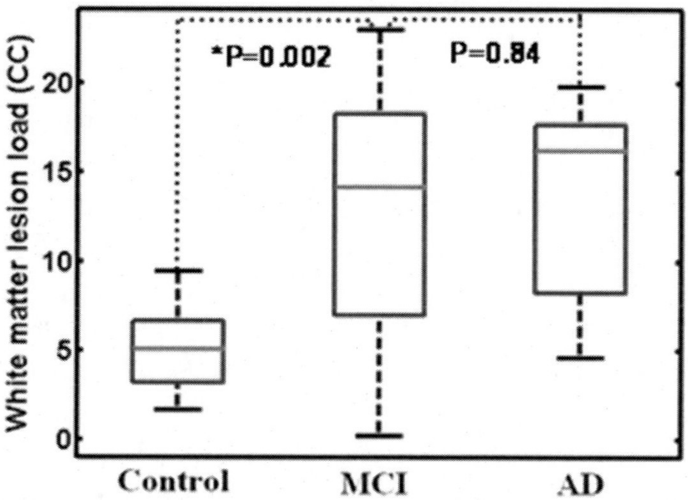

Source and color image: Adapted from Zhou Y, Yu F, Duong TQ, Alzheimer's Disease Neuroimaging Initiative (2015) White matter lesion load is associated with resting state functional MRI activity and amyloid PET but not FDG in mild cognitive impairment and early Alzheimer's disease patients. *J Magn Reson Imaging* 41:102-109. Used with permission.

Figure 2. Compared to controls, there was significantly increased whole brain white matter lesion load (WMLL in units of ml) in MCI and AD groups ($P = 0.002$) compared to controls. Note there was no significant difference of WMLL between MCI and early AD group. The boxes have lines at the lower quartile (horizontal blue lines), median (horizontal red lines), and upper quartile values. The whiskers are lines extending from each end of the boxes to show the extent of the rest of the data.

Based on the PET amyloid image (i.e., SUVR) (Figure 1b), patients with MCI (0.42±0.15) and early AD (1.58±0.20) patients showed a higher-degree of amyloid deposition compared to controls (0.15±0.12), both with $P < 0.001$. Regional normalized uptake values also demonstrated significantly higher uptake values in MCI and AD, with the highest degree in the AD group with $P < 0.001$, including the PCC ($P < 0.005$) (1.15±0.21 in controls, 1.56±0.33 in MCI and 1.77±0.41 in AD) and MPFC ($P < 0.005$) (1.20±0.35 in controls, 1.66±0.35 in MCI and 1.82±0.27 in AD). However, there was no significant difference in the amyloid uptake between the patients with early AD compared to MCI in either the entire cortex ($P = 0.07$), PCC ($P = 0.07$), or MPFC ($P = 0.39$) (Zhou et al. 2012a).

A significant correlation was found between WMLL and amyloid load averaged over the whole cerebral cortex in all three groups (Pearson $r = 0.46$, $P = 0.015$; Spearman rank $r = 0.46$, $P = 0.013$) (Figure 3). There were also significant correlations between WMLL and amyloid load in the PCC (Pearson $r = 0.4$, $P = 0.04$; Spearman rank $r = 0.43$, $P = 0.023$), as well as the MPFC (Pearson $r = 0.45$, $P = 0.018$, Spearman rank $r = 0.43$, $P = 0.023$). Regarding the FDG uptake, there was significantly lower cerebral FDG SUVR in MCI and AD patients compared controls ($P = 0.002$) (Figure 4a). A negative correlation between FDG uptake and amyloid load was noted in the 3 groups ($r = -0.57$, $P = 0.0006$) (Figure 4b). FDG uptake was not correlated significantly with either WMLL or RS-fMRI activity.

RS-fMRI results showed significantly reduced (corrected $P < 0.05$) DMN connectivity and altered fALFF activity in both MCI and AD groups. A significant correlation was found between WMLL and DMN connectivity strength ($r = 0.56$, $P = 0.02$), as well as between WMLL and fALFF activity values ($r = 0.63$, $P = 0.01$) in MCI patients.

A significant correlation was found between amyloid load of the whole cerebral cortex and lower fALFF activity value in AD patients (r = 0.64, P = 0.046) (Zhou et al. 2015).

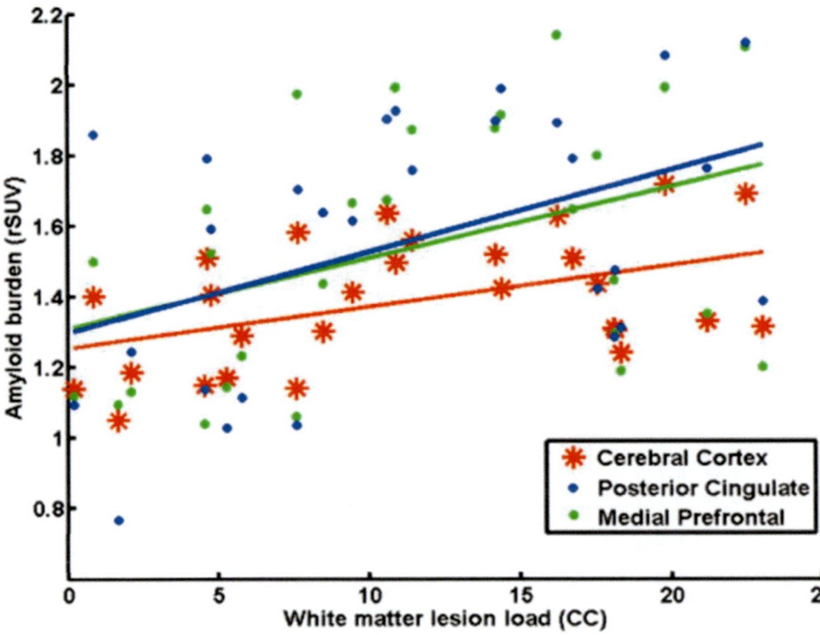

Source and color image: Adapted from Zhou Y, Yu F, Duong TQ, Alzheimer's Disease Neuroimaging Initiative (2015) White matter lesion load is associated with resting state functional MRI activity and amyloid PET but not FDG in mild cognitive impairment and early Alzheimer's disease patients. *J Magn Reson Imaging* 41:102-109. Used with permission.

Figure 3. There was significant correlation between white matter lesion load (WMLL) and amyloid load averaged over the whole brain cerebral cortex in all three groups, shown in red color (Pearson r = 0.46, P = 0.015; Spearman rank r = 0.46, P = 0.013). There were also significant correlations between WMLL and amyloid load in the posterior cingulate cortex (Pearson r = 0.4, P = 0.04; Spearman rank r = 0.43, P = 0.023) shown in blue color, as well as in the medial prefrontal cortex (Pearson r = 0.45, P = 0.018, Spearman rank r = 0.43, P = 0.023) (green color).

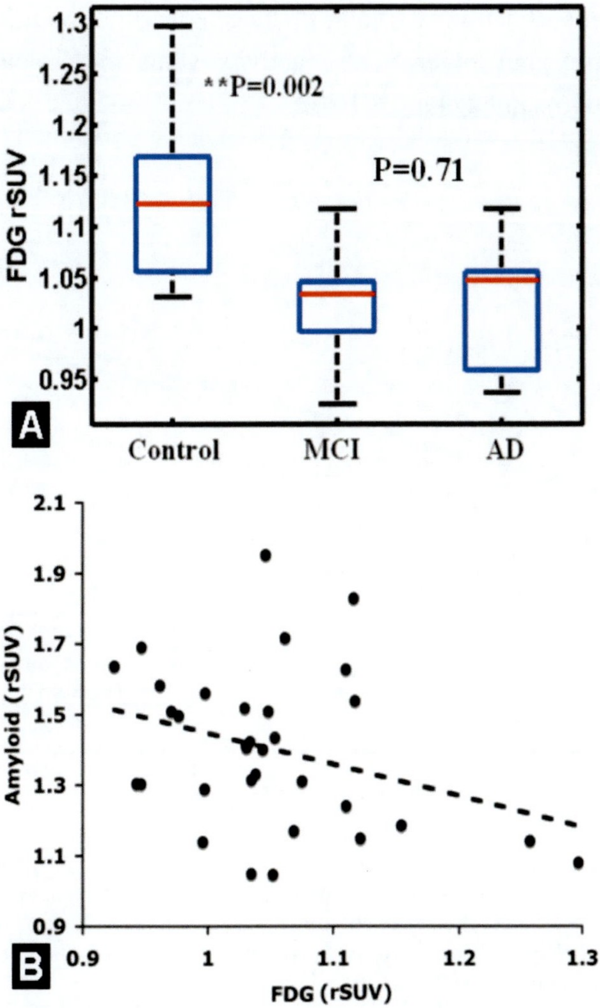

Source and color image: Adapted from Zhou Y, Yu F, Duong TQ, Alzheimer's Disease Neuroimaging Initiative (2015) White matter lesion load is associated with resting state functional MRI activity and amyloid PET but not FDG in mild cognitive impairment and early Alzheimer's disease patients. *J Magn Reson Imaging* 41:102-109. Used with permission.

Figure 4. A: Compared to controls, there was significantly decreased whole brain FDG standard uptake value ratio using cerebellum as reference region (rSUV) in MCI and AD groups (P = 0.002) compared to controls. Note there was no significant difference of FDG uptake between MCI and early AD group (P = 0.71). B: There was significant correlation between FDG uptake and amyloid load averaged over the whole brain cerebral cortex in all three groups (Pearson correlation r = -0.57, P = 0.0006).

4. Discussions and Conclusion

Our previous baseline findings indicate that tau images demonstrated expected higher deposition in the early possible pathological regions in hippocampal and temporal cortices (Zhou et al. 2017b). As expected and validated, quantitative Braak stage-based regional analyses showed highest tau deposition in the Braak stage II in the preclinical samples. Significant correlations were also found between tau and multiple MRI metrics including diffusion, perfusion and functional connectivity. Consistent with reported results, we observed significant PART effect including hippocampus and temporal cortex regions (Brier et al. 2016; Rodriguez-Vieitez et al. 2016; Schwarz et al. 2016). Furthermore, strong correlations were found between tau deposition in different sub-segments of temporal cortex and composite neurocognitive scores in the domain of memory and executive function from the ADNI data, as well as between regional tau and amyloid (mostly cortical regions), and between tau and FDG (including some sub-cortical regions). The PART effects observed in bilateral hippocampus and temporal cortices but not in other cortical regions confirm with recent tau pathological findings that PART-type pathology generally does not progress to the isocortical Braak stages and has limited extension beyond the temporal neocortex to other neocortical regions (Clavaguera et al. 2010). The quantitative SUV values were consistent with reported values in preclinical elderly samples, for instance, mean SUV = 1.18–1.19 for clinically normal individuals (Jack et al. 2016b). We also observed consistent regional tau distribution pattern and correlations with amyloid and FDG tracers (Vemuri et al. 2016). A recent study had reported voxel-wise focal negative correlations between [^{18}-F]THK5317 retention and [^{18}-F]FDG uptake, mainly in the frontal cortex, and focal positive correlations were found between [^{18}-F]THK5317 and [^{11}-C]PIB retentions isocortically (Chiotis et al. 2016). Our previous correlational result between PET tracers and memory tests was consistent with recent findings that tau was associated with decline in global cognition (Zhou, 2017a; Rodriguez-Vieitez et al. 2016). Significant correlations between tau and executive function composite score were found in our preclinical samples including frontal and amygdale regions as well as strong associations between tau in temporal cortex and executive function composite score in normal individuals (all $P < 0.01$). These results were consistent with the finding that worse performance on domain-specific neuropsychological tests was associated with greater [^{18}-F]-AV1451 uptake in key regions implicated in memory (medial temporal lobes), visuospatial function and language (Ossenkoppele et al. 2016).

In this study based on ADNI data, longitudinal tau changes (0.1-1.5% yearly rate of increment) demonstrated a posterior to anterior occipito-temporal degradation pattern at different follow-up times in comparison to baseline. The most significant progression of tau deposition was present in the Braak stage IV regions including temporal pole and middle temporal cortex. Decrement of tau deposition in the early transentorhinal region and fusiform at follow-ups could possibly due to the spreading effects from these earlier Braak stage regions (I & III) to relatively later stage regions such as temporal poles. Our results were consistent with the reported longitudinal changes with about 2.9% bi-yearly rate of cortical tau, especially in regions of medial/inferior temporal cortices at prodromal stage of AD (Cho et al. 2019). Significant longitudinal changes of regional amyloid SUVR deposition demonstrated about 0.3-0.4% beta-amyloid increment at 24-month follow-up times in the temporal cortex, especially in the middle and inferior temporal sub-segments, compared to baseline. The whole brain cerebrum had about 0.1% increment including regions of bilateral parsorbitalis (about 0.45% biyearly rate) and right lateral occipital cortex (0.15% rate) over 24 months. These results were in line with the recently published values of about 0.5% accumulation rate of amyloid in the preclinical stage0-1 samples (Guo et al. 2018; Gordon et al. 2016).

As for FDG glucose metabolism, longitudinal data presented significant reductions (most of $P \leq 0.0001$) of glucose metabolic rate at variable follow-up times in the regions of bilateral temporal, angular and posterior cortices. And the rate of FDG metabolism decline varied slightly for different regions, with about -1.6% every year decline of glucose metabolic rate for the posterior cingulum, -1.3% yearly for left temporal cortex and -1.9% yearly for bilateral angular region. The decline yearly rate of FDG was in agreement with the published 1-2 % hypometabolic rate in the temporoparietal regions (Caballero et al. 2015). Similar FDG hypometabolic degrees at follow-ups were observed for the median and mode metrics in these regions, indicating consistent longitudinal FDG hypometabolic changes. Furthermore, regional coherences were maintained (e.g., between hippocampus and other region) in the cortical regions for both tau and amyloid images using either SUVR or volumetry. Significant positive correlations between tau and amyloid as well as negative correlations between tau and FDG in several brain regions had been reported previously (Zhou 2017b). Our current longitudinal observations of similar rates of incremental tau but decremental FDG uptake indicated intracellular tau tangles and neurodegenerative hypometabolism were strongly associated, together with the slower amyloid progression in mostly preclinical samples. It had been reported that the rates of pathological tau and amyloid accumulation as well as metabolic decline increase from predromal to early AD stage (Landau et al. 2015).

Regarding WMH, we found a typical peri-ventricular and frontal WM lesion distribution in MCI and AD patients (Damian et al. 1994; Greicius et al. 2004; Bendfeldt et al. 2010). Our comparison results also showed significantly elevated global WMLL in MCI patients compared to controls. Meanwhile, these values were not significantly different for early AD compared to MCI patients. A recent study indicated that based on global and temporal WM lesions alone, differentiation between stages of cognitive impairment, as well as prediction of progression to dementia (including AD), may be achieved (Mortamais et al. 2013). Our results support the notion that WM lesions were detectable at a prodromal stage and may provide additional insights into early AD detection. On the other hand, there is no longitudinal change of global white matter hyperintensity at 3 to 24 months time interval compared to baseline ($P > 0.05$). Our results were in agreement with the observation that the severity of baseline WMH (for instance, only 0.02% longitudinal change in healthy controls) predicts the longitudinal progression of WMLL (Burton et al. 2008). The moderate correlation between WMLL and amyloid load in controls as well as affected populations suggests a possible link between microvascular damage and amyloid pathology at the early stages of Alzheimer disease (i.e., MCI and early AD). However, the spatial distribution patterns of WMLL (periventricular and frontal WM) and amyloid load (predominantly in MPFC and PCC cortical areas) were different, suggesting these two regions may be distinctly involved at different stages of dementia. A significant negative correlation was found between FDG uptake and amyloid load in the three aging populations, indicating a correspondence between amyloid pathology and metabolism (e.g., hypometabolism in MCI and AD patients) at the early stages of AD as well. The different temporal trajectories of FDG and Florbetapir has been reported before (Jack et al. 2013), and it might be possible that at early stages especially at MCI and AD, these two biomarkers co-occur and thus producing significant correlations. However we also noted the differences between these two tracers given that FDG is more sensitive in diagnosing AD (from mild to severe) while Florbetapir amyloid tracer is used for pathological specification and prediction of disease progression, particularly in early AD (Mosconi et al. 2010).

The Aβ deposition is assumed to be the "trigger" of the tau to cause the neurodegeneration in brain based on its earlier onset of pathological accumulation compared to the PHF-tau (Jack et al. 2013; Jack et al. 2016a). Whether PHF-tau can serve as an independent tracer for diagnosis different sub-types of dementia patients needs further investigation. One of the future directions would probably be to construct disease-specific tau distribution patterns including not only early AD (which is spatially more confined to medial temporal lobe, but also other types of dementia such as fronto-temporal dementia (Sarazin et al. 2016; Scholl et al. 2016). Although we only used static [18-F]-AV-1451 SUV values, recent kinetic analysis based on [18-F]-AV-1451 SUVR curves suggesting that an SUVR calculated over imaging window of 80-100 min (as currently used in clinical studies) provides estimates of PHF tau burden in good correlation with non-specific binding potential of tau (Barret et al. 2016).

Potential future work also includes adjustment for these confounding factors including clinical and genetic data and acquisition of more complete and multi-point longitudinal data to elucidate the causality effects of different imaging biomarkers (Lim et al. 2016; Smith et al. 2016). To improve the accuracy of the diagnosis of the tracer, reduction of the off-target binding of the tau tracer (e.g., subcortical striatal regions), and incorporating kinetic parametric results such as R1 and DVR similar to the amyloid imaging quantification at different disease population might help to further the interpretation of the subcortical to cortical tau spreading results (Barret et al. 2016; Chiotis et al. 2016; Lockhart et al. 2016; Wang et al. 2016). It has been suggested that tau spreading in other isocortical regions required the presence of cortical Aβ (Prashanthi and Petersen, 2016; Rodriguez-Vieitez et al. 2016).

Taken together, tau, amyloid, FDG and associated WMH are pathological hallmarks of AD. The concurrence of WM hyperintensity, GM atrophy, structural disconnectivity and functional hyper-perfusion and the higher tau, amyloid and lower FDG uptake in entorhinal, hippocampal and other temporal regions suggested detectable pathological, structural and functional brain changes at both molecular and macroscopic levels, at even early stages of dementia including MCI patients. Our longitudinal results indicated variable degrees of changes of different imaging biomarkers at follow-ups compared to baseline.

Especially higher tau deposition and FDG hypometabolism with similar neurodegenerative rates but slower amyloid accumulation (at a slower rate than tau and FDG, possibly due to the earlier onset of amyloid plaques of extracellular progression) were observed with molecular imaging techniques. However, no significant or slow WMH progression was found over 1-3 year follow-up time and no significant difference between MCI and early AD, possibly due to the distinct pathophysiology of this microvascular risk factor. A complete longitudinal data of all the imaging biomarkers including tau, amyloid, FDG, WMH, functional and structural connectivity, hippocampal volume and some newly developed imaging metrics for quantitative inflammation and myelin maps in the near future would help elucidate the causality and connections among different neuropathological burdens and underlying functional as well as microstructural changes.

ACKNOWLEGEMENTS

Data collection and sharing for this project was funded by the Alzheimer's Disease Neuroimaging Initiative (ADNI) (National Institutes of Health Grant U01 AG024904) and DOD ADNI (Department of Defense award number W81XWH-12-2-0012). ADNI is funded by the National Institute on Aging, the National Institute of Biomedical Imaging and Bioengineering, and through generous contributions from the following: AbbVie, Alzheimer's Association; Alzheimer's Drug Discovery Foundation; Araclon Biotech; BioClinica, Inc.; Biogen; Bristol-Myers Squibb Company; CereSpir, Inc.; Cogstate; Eisai Inc.; Elan Pharmaceuticals, Inc.; Eli Lilly and Company; EuroImmun; F. Hoffmann-La Roche Ltd and its affiliated company Genentech, Inc.; Fujirebio; GE Healthcare; IXICO Ltd.; Janssen Alzheimer Immunotherapy Research and Development, LLC.; Johnson and Johnson Pharmaceutical Research and Development LLC.;

Lumosity; Lundbeck; Merck and Co., Inc.; Meso Scale Diagnostics, LLC.; NeuroRx Research; Neurotrack Technologies; Novartis Pharmaceuticals Corporation; Pfizer Inc.; Piramal Imaging; Servier; Takeda Pharmaceutical Company; and Transition Therapeutics. The Canadian Institutes of Health Research is providing funds to support ADNI clinical sites in Canada. Private sector contributions are facilitated by the Foundation for the National Institutes of Health (www.fnih.org). The grantee organization is the Northern California Institute for Research and Education, and the study is coordinated by the Alzheimer's Therapeutic Research Institute at the University of Southern California. ADNI data are disseminated by the Laboratory for NeuroImaging at the University of Southern California.

REFERENCES

[1] Ariza M, Kolb HC, Moechars D, Rombouts F, Andres JI (2015) Tau Positron Emission Tomography (PET) Imaging: Past, Present, and Future. *J Med Chem* 58:4365-4382.

[2] Barret O, Alagille D, Sanabria S, Comley RA, Weimer RM, Borroni E, Mintun M, Seneca N, Papin C, Morley T, Marek K, Seibyl JP, Tamagnan GD, Jennings D (2016) Kinetic Modeling of the Tau PET Tracer 18F-AV-1451 in Human Healthy Volunteers and Alzheimer's Disease Subjects. *J Nucl Med.*

[3] Bendfeldt K, Blumhagen JO, Egger H, Loetscher P, Denier N, Kuster P, Traud S, Mueller-Lenke N, Naegelin Y, Gass A, Hirsch J, Kappos L, Nichols TE, Radue EW, Borgwardt SJ (2010) Spatiotemporal distribution pattern of white matter lesion volumes and their association with regional grey matter volume reductions in relapsing-remitting multiple sclerosis. *Human brain mapping* 31:1542-1555.

[4] Braak H, Braak E (1991) Neuropathological stageing of Alzheimer-related changes. *Acta neuropathologica* 82:239-259.

[5] Brendel M, Jaworska A, Probst F, Overhoff F, Korzhova V, Lindner S, Carlsen J, Bartenstein P, Harada R, Kudo Y, Haass C, Van Leuven F, Okamura N, Herms J, Rominger A (2016) Small-Animal PET Imaging of Tau Pathology with 18F-THK5117 in 2 Transgenic Mouse Models. *J Nucl Med* 57:792-798.

[6] Brickman AM, Provenzano FA, Muraskin J, Manly JJ, Blum S, Apa Z, Stern Y, Brown TR, Luchsinger JA, Mayeux R (2012) Regional white matter hyperintensity volume, not hippocampal atrophy, predicts incident Alzheimer disease in the community. *Archives of neurology* 69:1621-1627.

[7] Brier MR, Gordon B, Friedrichsen K, McCarthy J, Stern A, Christensen J, Owen C, Aldea P, Su Y, Hassenstab J, Cairns NJ, Holtzman DM, Fagan AM, Morris JC, Benzinger TL, Ances BM (2016) Tau and Abeta imaging, CSF measures, and cognition in Alzheimer's disease. *Sci Transl Med* 8:338ra366.

[8] Buckner RL, Snyder AZ, Shannon BJ, LaRossa G, Sachs R, Fotenos AF, Sheline YI, Klunk WE, Mathis CA, Morris JC, Mintun MA (2005) Molecular, structural, and functional characterization of Alzheimer's disease: evidence for a relationship between default activity, amyloid, and memory. *The Journal of neuroscience*: the official journal of the Society for Neuroscience 25:7709-7717.

[9] Burton EJ, McKeith IG, Burn DJ, Firbank MJ, O'Brien JT (2006) Progression of white matter hyperintensities in Alzheimer disease, dementia with lewy bodies, and Parkinson disease dementia: a comparison with normal aging, *Am J Geriatr Psychiatry* 14(10):842-9.

[10] Caballero MÁ , Brendel M, Delker A, Ren J, Rominger A, Bartenstein P, Dichgans M, Weiner MW, Ewers M; Alzheimer's Disease Neuroimaging Initative (ADNI) (2015) Map-ping 3-year

changes in gray matter and metabolism in Aβ-positive nondemented subjects. *Neurobiol. Aging* 36(11):2913-2924.

[11] Chiotis K, Saint-Aubert L, Savitcheva I, Jelic V, Andersen P, Jonasson M, Eriksson J, Lubberink M, Almkvist O, Wall A, Antoni G, Nordberg A (2016) Imaging in-vivo tau pathology in Alzheimer's disease with THK5317 PET in a multimodal paradigm. *Eur J Nucl Med Mol Imaging* 43:1686-1699.

[12] Cho H, Choi JY, Lee HS, Lee JH, Ryu YH, Lee MS, Jack CR Jr, Lyoo CH (2019) Progres-sive tau accumulation in Alzheimer's disease: two-year follow-up study. *J Nucl Med.* doi: 10.2967/jnumed.118.221697.

[13] Clavaguera F, Goedert M, Tolnay M (2010) [Induction and spreading of tau pathology in a mouse model of Alzheimer's disease]. *Med Sci* (Paris) 26:121-124.

[14] Damian MS, Schilling G, Bachmann G, Simon C, Stoppler S, Dorndorf W (1994) White matter lesions and cognitive deficits: relevance of lesion pattern? *Acta neurologica Scandinavica* 90:430-436.

[15] Debette S, Markus HS (2010) The clinical importance of white matter hyperintensities on brain magnetic resonance imaging: systematic review and meta-analysis. *BMJ* 341:c3666.

[16] Geppert AM, Wroblewska KA, Przedpelska-Ober EM (2007) Greater frequency of subcortical lesions in severely demented patients with early onset Alzheimer's disease. *Alzheimer's & dementia*: the journal of the Alzheimer's Association 3:54-57.

[17] Gordon BA, Blazey T, Su Y, Fagan AM, Holtzman DM, Morris JC, Tammie L. S. Benzinger TLS (2016) Longitudinal β-Amyloid Deposition and Hippocampal Volume in Preclinical Alzheimer Disease and Suspected Non–Alzheimer Disease Pathophysiology. *JAMA Neurol.* 73(10): 1192–1200.

[18] Greicius MD, Krasnow B, Reiss AL, Menon V (2004) Functional connectivity in the resting brain: a network analysis of the default mode hypothesis. *Proc Natl Aca Sci* U S A 101:4637-4642.

[19] Guo T, Dukart J, Brendel M, Rominger A, Grimmer T, Yakushev I (2018) Rate of β-amyloid accumulation varies with baseline amyloid burden: Implications for anti-amyloid drug trials. *Alzheimer's & Dementia* 14:1387-1396.

[20] Holmes HE et al. (2016) Imaging the accumulation and suppression of tau pathology using multiparametric MRI. *Neurobiol Aging* 39:184-194.

[21] Jack CR, Jr., Knopman DS, Jagust WJ, Petersen RC, Weiner M, Alsen PS, Shaw LM, Vermuri P, Wiste HJ, Welgand SD, Lesnick TG, Pankratz VS, Donohue MC, Trojanowski JQ (2013) Tracking pathophysiological processes in Alzheimer's disease: an updated hypothetical model of dynamic biomarkers. *Lancet neurology* 12:207-216.

[22] Jack CR, Jr., Knopman DS, Jagust WJ, Shaw LM, Aisen PS, Weiner MW, Petersen RC, Trojanowski JQ (2010) Hypothetical model of dynamic biomarkers of the Alzheimer's pathological cascade. *Lancet Neurol* 9:119-128.

[23] Jack CR, Jr., Bennett DA, Blennow K, Carrillo MC, Feldman HH, Frisoni GB, Hampel H, Jagust WJ, Johnson KA, Knopman DS, Petersen RC, Scheltens P, Sperling RA, Dubois B (2016a) A/T/N: An unbiased descriptive classification scheme for Alzheimer disease biomarkers. *Neurology* 87:539-547.

[24] Jack CR, Jr., Wiste HJ, Weigand SD, Therneau TM, Lowe VJ, Knopman DS, Gunter JL, Senjem ML, Jones DT, Kantarci K, Machulda MM, Mielke MM, Roberts RO, Vemuri P, Reyes DA, Petersen RC (2016b) Defining imaging biomarker cut points for brain aging and Alzheimer's disease. *Alzheimer's Dement*.

[25] Kahlson MA, Colodner KJ (2015) Glial Tau Pathology in Tauopathies: Functional Consequences. *J Exp Neurosci* 9:43-50.

[26] Landau SM, Fero A, Baker SL, Koeppe R, Mintun M, Chen K, Reiman EM, Jagust WJ (2015) Measurement of longitudinal β-amyloid change with 18F-florbetapir PET and standardized uptake value ratios, *J Nucl Med*. 56(4):567-74.

[27] Leuzy A., Rodriguez-Vieitez E., Saint-Aubert L., Chiotis K., Almkvist O., Savitcheva I., Jonasson M., Lubberink M., Wall A., Antoni G., Nordberg A., Longitudinal uncoupling of cerebral perfusion, glucose metabolism, and tau deposition in Alzheimer's disease, *Alzheimers Dement*. 2018; 14(5):652-663.

[28] Lim YY et al. (2016) BDNF Val66Met moderates memory impairment, hippocampal function and tau in preclinical autosomal dominant Alzheimer's disease. *Brain* 139:2766-2777.

[29] Lockhart SN, Baker SL, Okamura N, Furukawa K, Ishiki A, Furumoto S, Tashiro M, Yanai K, Arai H, Kudo Y, Harada R, Tomita N, Hiraoka K, Watanuki S, Jagust WJ (2016) Dynamic PET Measures of Tau Accumulation in Cognitively Normal Older Adults and Alzheimer's Disease Patients Measured Using [18F] THK-5351. *PLoS One* 11:e0158460.

[30] Lowe VJ, Curran G, Fang P, Liesinger AM, Josephs KA, Parisi JE, Kantarci K, Boeve BF, Pandey MK, Bruinsma T, Knopman DS, Jones DT, Petrucelli L, Cook CN, Graff-Radford NR, Dickson DW, Petersen RC, Jack CR, Jr., Murray ME (2016) An autoradiographic evaluation of AV-1451 Tau PET in dementia. *Acta Neuropathol Commun* 4:58.

[31] Mikheev A, Nevsky G, Govindan S, Grossman R, Rusinek H (2008) Fully automatic segmentation of the brain from T1-weighted MRI using Bridge Burner algorithm. *Journal of magnetic resonance imaging: JMRI* 27:1235-1241.

[32] Moghekar A, Kraut M, Elkins W, Troncoso J, Zonderman AB, Resnick SM, O'Brien RJ (2012) Cerebral white matter disease is associated with Alzheimer pathology in a prospective cohort. *Alzheimer's & dementia*: the journal of the Alzheimer's Association 8:S71-77.

[33] Mortamais M, Reynes C, Brickman AM, Provenzano FA, Muraskin J, Portet F, Berr C, Touchon J, Bonafe A, le Bars E, Maller JJ, Meslin C, Sabatier R, Ritchie K, Artero S (2013) Spatial distribution of cerebral white matter lesions predicts

progression to mild cognitive impairment and dementia. *PloS One* 8:e56972.

[34] Mosconi L, Berti V, Glodzik L, Pupi A, De Santi S, de Leon MJ (2010) Pre-Clinical Detection of Alzheimer's Disease Using FDG-PET, with or without Amyloid Imaging. *Journal of Alzheimer's Disease* 20:843-854.

[35] Nordahl CW, Ranganath C, Yonelinas AP, DeCarli C, Fletcher E, Jagust WJ (2006) White Matter Changes Compromise Prefrontal Cortex Function in Healthy Elderly Individuals. *Journal of Cognitive Neuroscience* 18:418-429.

[36] Ossenkoppele R, Schonhaut DR, Scholl M, Lockhart SN, Ayakta N, Baker SL, O'Neil JP, Janabi M, Lazaris A, Cantwell A, Vogel J, Santos M, Miller ZA, Bettcher BM, Vossel KA, Kramer JH, Gorno-Tempini ML, Miller BL, Jagust WJ, Rabinovici GD (2016) Tau PET patterns mirror clinical and neuroanatomical variability in Alzheimer's disease. *Brain* 139:1551-1567.

[37] Patel MJ, Boada FE, Price JC, Sheu LK, Tudorascu DL, Reynolds Iii CF, Aizenstein HJ (2012) Association of small vessel ischemic white matter changes with BOLD fMRI imaging in the elderly. *Psychiatry research* 204:117-122.

[38] Prashanthi V LV, Knopman DS, Senjem ML, Kemp KJ, Schwarz CG, Przybelski SA, Machuldad MM,, Petersen RC JC (2016) Tau-PET uptake: Regional variation in average SUVR and impact of amyloid deposition. *Alzheimer's & Dementia*: Diagnosis, Assessment & Disease Monitoring:1-10.

[39] Reed BR, Marchant NL, Jagust WJ, Decarli C, Mack W, Chui HC (2012) Coronary risk corrlates with cerebral amyloid deposition. *Neurobiology of aging* 33:1979-1987.

[40] Rodriguez-Vieitez E, Saint-Aubert L, Carter SF, Almkvist O, Farid K, Scholl M, Chiotis K, Thordardottir S, Graff C, Wall A, Langstrom B, Nordberg A (2016) Diverging longitudinal changes in astrocytosis and amyloid PET in autosomal dominant Alzheimer's disease. *Brain* 139:922-936.

[41] Ryan NS, Keihaninejad S, Shakespeare TJ, Lehmann M, Crutch SJ, Malone IB, Thornton JS, Mancini L, Hyare H, Yousy T, Ridgway GR, Zhang H, Modat M, Alexander DC, Rossor MN, Ourselin S, Fox NC (2011) Magnetic resonance imaging evidence for presymptomatic change in thalamus and caudate in familial Alzheimer's disease. *Brain: a journal of neurology* 136:1399-1414.

[42] Salat DH, Tuch DS, Greve DN, van der Kouwe AJW, Hevelone ND, Zaleta AK, Rosen BR, Fischl B, Corkin S, Rosas HD, Dale AM (2005) Age-related alterations in white matter microstructure measured by diffusion tensor imaging. *Neurobiology of aging* 26:1215-1227.

[43] Sarazin M, Lagarde J, Bottlaender M (2016) Distinct tau PET imaging patterns in typical and atypical Alzheimer's disease. *Brain* 139:1321-1324.

[44] Scholl M, Lockhart SN, Schonhaut DR, O'Neil JP, Janabi M, Ossenkoppele R, Baker SL, Vogel JW, Faria J, Schwimmer HD, Rabinovici GD, Jagust WJ (2016) PET Imaging of Tau Deposition in the Aging Human Brain. *Neuron* 89:971-982.

[45] Schwarz AJ, Yu P, Miller BB, Shcherbinin S, Dickson J, Navitsky M, Joshi AD, Devous MD, Sr., Mintun MS (2016) Regional profiles of the candidate tau PET ligand 18F-AV-1451 recapitulate key features of Braak histopathological stages. *Brain* 139:1539-1550.

[46] Shcherbinin S, Schwarz AJ, Joshi A, Navitsky M, Flitter M, Shankle WR, Devous MD, Sr., Mintun MA (2016) Kinetics of the Tau PET Tracer 18F-AV-1451 (T807) in Subjects with Normal Cognitive Function, Mild Cognitive Impairment, and Alzheimer Disease. *J Nucl Med* 57:1535-1542.

[47] Silverman DH et al. (2001) Positron emission tomography in evaluation of dementia: Regional brain metabolism and long-term outcome. *JAMA*: The journal of the American Medical Association 286:2120-2127.

[48] Smith R, Puschmann A, Scholl M, Ohlsson T, van Swieten J, Honer M, Englund E, Hansson O (2016) 18F-AV-1451 tau PET imaging correlates strongly with tau neuropathology in MAPT mutation carriers. *Brain* 139:2372-2379.

[49] Sperling R, Mormino E, Johnson K (2014) The evolution of preclinical Alzheimer's disease: implications for prevention trials. *Neuron* 84:608-622.

[50] Takada LT, Camiz P, Grinberg LT, da Costa Leite C (2009) Non-inflammatory cerebral amyloid angiopathy as a cause of rapidly progressive dementia - a case study. *Dementia Neuropsychology* 3:352-257.

[51] Villemagne VL, Okamura N (2014) In vivo tau imaging: obstacles and progress. *Alzheimers Dement* 10:S254-264.

[52] Villemagne VL, Okamura N (2016) Tau imaging in the study of ageing, Alzheimer's disease, and other neurodegenerative conditions. *Curr Opin Neurobiol* 36:43-51.

[53] Wang L, Benzinger TL, Su Y, Christensen J, Friedrichsen K, Aldea P, McConathy J, Cairns NJ, Fagan AM, Morris JC, Ances BM (2016) Evaluation of Tau Imaging in Staging Alzheimer Disease and Revealing Interactions Between beta-Amyloid and Tauopathy. *JAMA Neurol* 73:1070-1077.

[54] Wardlaw JM, Smith EE, Biessels GJ, et al. (2013) Neuroimaging standards for research into small vessel disease and its contribution to ageing and neurodegeneration. *Lancet neurology* 12:822-838.

[55] Wells JA et al. (2015) In vivo imaging of tau pathology using multi-parametric quantitative MRI. *Neuroimage* 111:369-378.

[56] Whitwell JL, Jack CR, Jr., Duffy JR, Strand EA, Gunter JL, Senjem ML, Murphy MC, Kantarci K, Machulda MM, Lowe VJ, Josephs KA (2013) Microbleeds in the logopenic variant of primary progressive aphasia. *Alzheimer's & Dementia* 9:1-5.

[57] Xia C, Dickerson BC (2016) Tau PET: the next frontier in molecular imaging of dementia. *Int Psychogeriatr*:1-4.

[58] Zhou Y, Dougherty JH, Jr., Hubner KF, Bai B, Cannon RL, Hutson RK (2008) Abnormal connectivity in the posterior cingulate and hippocampus in early Alzheimer's disease and mild cognitive impairment. *Alzheimers Dement* 4:265-270.

[59] Zhou Y, Ge Y, De Leon M (2012a) White matter lesion load is associated with resting state fMRI activity in mild cognitive impairment patients. *Alzheimer's & Dementia* 8:535-536.

[60] Zhou Y, Sojkova J, Resnick SM, Wong DF (2012b) Relative equilibrium plot improves graphical analysis and allows bias correction of standardized uptake value ratio in quantitative 11C-PiB PET studies. *J Nucl Med* 53:622-628.

[61] Zhou Y, Lui YW (2013) Small-World Properties in Mild Cognitive Impairment and Early Alzheimer's Disease: A Cortical Thickness MRI Study. ISRN *Geriatr* 2013.

[62] Zhou Y, Yu F, Duong TQ, Alzheimer's Disease Neuroimaging Initiative (2015) White matter lesion load is associated with resting state functional MRI activity and amyloid PET but not FDG in mild cognitive impairment and early Alzheimer's disease patients. *J Magn Reson Imaging* 41:102-109.

[63] Zhou Y (2016a) *Functional Neuroimaging with Multiple Modalities:* Nova Publishers.

[64] Zhou Y (2016b) Quantitative PET/MRI Evaluation and Application in Dementia. *Jacobs J Med Diagn Med Imaging* 1(1).

[65] Zhou Y, Bai B. and ADNI (2017) Tau and Other PET/MRI Imaging Biomarkers for Detecting and Diagnosing Early Dementia. *Jacobs J Med Diagn Med Imaging* 2(1):017.

Chapter 5

MULTI-PARAMETRIC EVIDENCES AND HORIZON IN METABOLISM AND AGING

ABSTRACT

Maintaining good metabolic profile plays a significant role in improving the quality of life at aging. Widely recommended physical and psychological strategies include exercise, calorie restriction (such as healthy diet), anti-aging neuroprotective and anti-inflammation therapy. Most occurring risks at middle age range ([45-65] years old) are obesity, insulin resistance, inflammation, alterations in the hypothalamus-hypophysis suprarenal axis activity, stress and hypertension that could increase the prevalence of metabolic syndrome. Metabolic syndrome increases with age and particularly for women. Significant associations were seen between imaging measures and cardiovascular risk factors at both baseline and 18-month follow-ups. An example of significant correlations between longitudinal MRI vascular reactivity parameter-hyperemia duration and cardiovascular biomarkers including high-density cholesterol, C-reactive protein, triglycerides and body mass index is given. Physical exercise, healthy diet and calorie restriction therapy as well as arts training could be some promising prevention strategies to reduce and modify the atherosclerosis and cardiovascular risks, as well as help preserve working memory and executive function at aging. Together with accurate imaging guidance, early detection and treatment could be achieved with the ultimate goal of improving quality of life at middle age and extending longevity.

HORIZON IN METABOLISM AND AGING

Associated with the aging-related brain changes are the cognitive deterioration usually in the domains of episodic memory, working memory and executive function. We had reported reduction of default-mode network functional connectivity together with increased compensation of dorsal attentional network, suggesting of decreasing executive function reserve (Zhou 2016). Aside from individual health conditions, a number of social-environmental factors also contribute to the decline of cognitive function due to the accumulation of oxidative stress, inflammatory reactions and cardio-vascular risks (de la Torre 2016). Metabolic abnormality is one of the common middle-age (range about 45-65 years, American Psychiatric Association, DSM-IV 1994) risk factors including glucose hypo-metabolism and insulin tolerance increases (Lewis and Keshari 2018). The imbalance and dysregulation of the energy delivery/consumption could lead to diabetes, neurodegenerative disease and cardiac dysfunction overtime without timely cure and treatment (Raz et al. 2005).

While the brain gains experience, wisdom and memory with aging, metabolic and cardiovascular physiological challenges are also present. Cross-sectional aging gradients with largely decline of perceptual speed, reasoning, memory, knowledge, language fluency and intellectual abilities were found with age range of [25-100] years old (Baltes et al. 1997). Most occurring risks at middle age range [45-65] years old are obesity, insulin resistance, inflammation, changes in the activity of the hypothalamus-hypophysis suprarenal axis, stress and hypertension that could increase the prevalence of metabolic syndrome. A cluster of these pathophysiological abnormalities, especially obesity, insulin resistance, impaired glucose tolerance, dyslipidemia and high blood pressure, are interconnected and called metabolic syndrome (Bonomini et al. 2015).

Based on the World Health Organization definition and published research, metabolic syndrome is defined as following: the presence of any one of these three conditions including diabetes mellitus, impaired glucose tolerance, impaired fasting glucose or insulin resistance; and together with two of the following four biomarker metrics: a. Blood pressure ≥ 140/90 mmHg; b. Dyslipidemia triglycerides (TG) ≥1.695 mmol/L with high-density lipoprotein cholesterol (HDL-C) ≤ 0.9 mmol/L (for male) and ≤ 1.0 mmol/L (for female); c. Central obesity; ratio of waist to hip >0.90 (for male) and >0.85 (for female), or body mass index (BMI) >30 kg/m^2; and d. Microalbuminuria with urinary albumin excretion ratio ≥ 20 μg/min or the ratio of albumin to creatinine ≥30 mg/g (World Health Organization 1999; Alberti and Zimmet 1999; Aguilar-Salinas et al. 2003).

Metabolic syndrome increases with age, with about 46.7% among those aged 60 years, 60% of the US population older than 50, compared to about 18.3% among those aged 20-39 years. Women has higher prevalence than men (about 5% higher, P<0.001), and highest prevalence in Hispanics race (35%) (Ford et al. 2002). In patients with coronary artery disease (CAD), 50% have metabolic syndrome. Particularly for women, metabolic abnormalities increases even after age-adjustment, when four following risks present to increase the prevalence: 58% for abdominal obesity, 28% for hypertriglyceridemia, 37% for high blood pressure, and 29% for fasting glucose (Ford et al. 2004; Churilla et al. 2007; Mozumdar et al. 2011).

It is well known that maintaining good metabolic profile plays a significant role in improving the quality of life at aging. Widely recommended physical and psychological strategies include exercise, calorie restriction (such as healthy diet), anti-aging neuro-protection and anti-inflammation therapies. Arts training had showed improvements of brain neuroplasticity and enhanced neuronal activity in certain brain function including executive function, high-level cognitive and communication functions as illustrated with neuroimaging MRI and PET modalities (Rizzo et al. 2018). After arts therapies, such as music, painting, and writing, elderly participants presented better cognitive functions in domains of memory and attention, social function such as self-confidence as well as neuropsychological effects with reduced agitation, depression and stress (Lindauer 2003; Gullette 2004). These arts training therapies also help older patients and the caregivers with their diminished abilities due to some complications at age such as stroke, trauma and Alzheimer's disease (AD) (Cohen 2006; Stern 2009).

Exercise (especially aerobic and long-term physical activity) and regular physical activity also plays an active role in brain functionality as reported by some studies. For instance, after regular exercise, brain circuits of dorsolateral prefrontal cortex and limbic structure were more active indicating benefits with relaxed emotion (happiness, relief and anti-depression) and improved attention, executive and cognitive brain functions (Boecker et al. 2012). During strenuous exercise, researchers also found decreased metabolic rate of glucose consumption with compensated lactate utilization in response to energy demand (Kemppainen et al. 2005).

Calorie restriction (CR), similar to the exercise effects, showed lower levels of metabolic rate with less reactive oxygen species and reduced oxidative damage (i.e., higher anti-inflammation effects) (Sohal and Weindruch 1996; Everitt et al. 2010). Apparently, there is a balance between the metabolizing energy reduction following CR and metabolic adaptation at tolerable and healthy levels (Redman et al. 2008). Animal studies found that CR reduces energy metabolism and oxidative stress to DNA, which could possibly help extend the lifespan (Redman and Ravussin 2007; Speakman 2004). Only 6 months of CR significantly lower cardiovascular risk factors (~28% lower), especially with lower triacylglycerol and higher HDL-cholesterol (Lefevre et al. 2009; Redman et al. 2009). CR also improved metabolic normality with reduced insulin resistance and β-cell dysfunction by reducing fat mass, delaying onsets of age-associated middle-life diseases such as Type-2 diabetes and obesity (Everitt et al. 2010). Detecting β-cell mass (BCM) abnormalities at early stages in response to the immune system attack in vivo is challenging which required both higher and full-spectrum dynamic spatiotemporal resolution as well as whole-body coverage and anatomic-functional penetration of imaging techniques (Lewis and Keshari 2018).

It has been generally accepted that the main underlying pathogenic mechanism of metabolic syndrome is the insulin resistance, and the secondary chronic inflammation and oxidative stress abnormalities. When presented together, these ill conditions could drive to morbidity and mortality at aging (Grundy et al. 2004; Morley 2004). Neuroprotective mechanisms such as glial cell and astrocytes activation for anti-inflammation, prevention of further disease progression and neuronal damage, as well as maintenance of axonal integrity and endothelial function, are widely used. Regarding treatment effects, it had been reported that short-term prevastatin treatment reduced myocardial infarct size in hypercholesterolemic rabbits, and rosuvastatin elevated antioxidant enzymes expression and HDL with lower oxidative stress (Everitt et al. 2010).

Longevity genes such as silent information regulator sirtuins, p66Shc, and mTOR could increase risks of metabolic syndrome. Glucose regulation and nutrition during longevity include insulin level, and IGF-1 signaling, as well as FOXO transcription factors play important roles (Everitt et al. 2010). In the long term, optimizing life style and enhancing mental activity with healthy metabolic profile including cholesterol and sterol regulatory element-binding protein (SREBP) are beneficial to early prevention of metabolic syndrome and protection against age-related neurological diseases (Rizzo et al. 2018). Physical exercise, healthy diet and calorie restriction therapies as well as arts training could be some promising prevention strategies to reduce and modify the atherosclerosis and cardiovascular risks, as well as help preserve working memory and executive function at aging (Menec 2003). Together with accurate imaging guidance, early detection and treatment could be achieved with the ultimate goal of improving quality of life at earlier age and extending longevity.

IMAGING EVIDENCE AND CORRELATIONS AMONG MULTIPLE PARAMETERS

Investigation the underlying pathophysiology mechanisms of diabetes with previously mentioned early prevention and intervention strategies using advanced diagnosing tools such as MRI and PET imaging techniques could help permanent cure of diabetes that usually relies on expensive medications and lifestyle change to maintain proper glucose regulation and insulin homeostasis (Bales et al. 2015; Fratiglioni 2004). Multi-modality imaging nowadays could be used to map multiple pathophysiological processes with age and brain changes affected with various risk factors simultaneously at early stage and with high spatiotemporal resolution (Zhou 2017; Zhou 2018).

Metabolic risk such as hypertension was reported to mediate aging effects based on MRI diffusion tensor imaging (DTI) metrics of fractional anisotropy (FA) and axial diffusivity (AX) that measures especially demyelination in corpus callosum body and dorsal cingulum with longitudinal studies (Bender et al. 2015). And even a clinically unremarkable elevation in metabolic syndrome risk affects and predicts the white matter deterioration within a relatively narrow time window (e.g., higher risks, lower FAs in young participants). We also found with in-house data that in participants with higher comorbidity indices (present with two or more diseases), significant negative correlations between FA in the active brain regions and age were observed ($r=-0.29 \sim -0.45$, $P \leq 0.001$) in response to the working memory and face recognition fMRI task. The aging trajectories of DTI parameters including FA, radial diffusivity (RD) and AX were slightly different from the normal participants (e.g., lower FA), but with significant higher FA in the positive active regions than the deactive brain regions identified with fMRI in these patients.

Comorbidity increases with age, including amyloid and tau deposition, diabetes, heart attack and obesity. It had been reported that the frequency of amyloid positive and neurodegeneration increased from age 65 years, and reached about 42% by age 89. The population frequency of single pathological burden however drops at old age, with 24% for neurodegeneration only and 17% for amyloidosis only by age 89 (Jack et al. 2014). Hypertension and obesity also moderate the relationships between beta-amyloid and cognitive decline; for instance, verbal learning and memory decline faster with both elevated beta-amyloid and risk factors present together (Clark et al. 2018). Recent metabolomics study found that sphingomyelins and ether-containing phosphatidylcholines were altered in preclinical AD stages, and acylcarnitines, branched-chain aminoacid valine as well as α-aminoadipic acid were modified in symptomatic stages (Toledo et al. 2017). Hypertensive participants had demonstrated shrinkages of hippocampus with age based on longitudinal volumetry (Raz et al. 2005).

Diabetes is associated with cerebrovascular risk including increased brain infarcts, with odds ration of 1.57 and $P < 0.0001$ (Abner et al. 2016). Although no Alzheimer's disease neuropathology found, when both diabetes and brain infarcts were presented, cognitive score was lower. And mini-mental state examination (MMSE) memory score was lower in cases of comorbid diabetes and Alzheimer's disease.

In our previous study, at baseline, significant associations were also observed between imaging measures and cardiovascular risk factors. For instance, all pulse wave velocity (PWV) metrics correlated with systolic blood pressure (SBP) ($r = 0.27$-0.42, $P < 0.001$). In non-smokers, the BMI and C-reactive protein levels correlated with microvascular MRI parameters, including forward flow time, hyperemia index, pulse ratio as well as overshoot, upslope and washout time (|r| = 0.16 – 0.97, P < 0.05). Further, total PWV correlated with cumulative cigarette smoke exposure expressed in terms of pack years in smokers (r = 0.52, P < 0.001) (Langham et al. 2015).

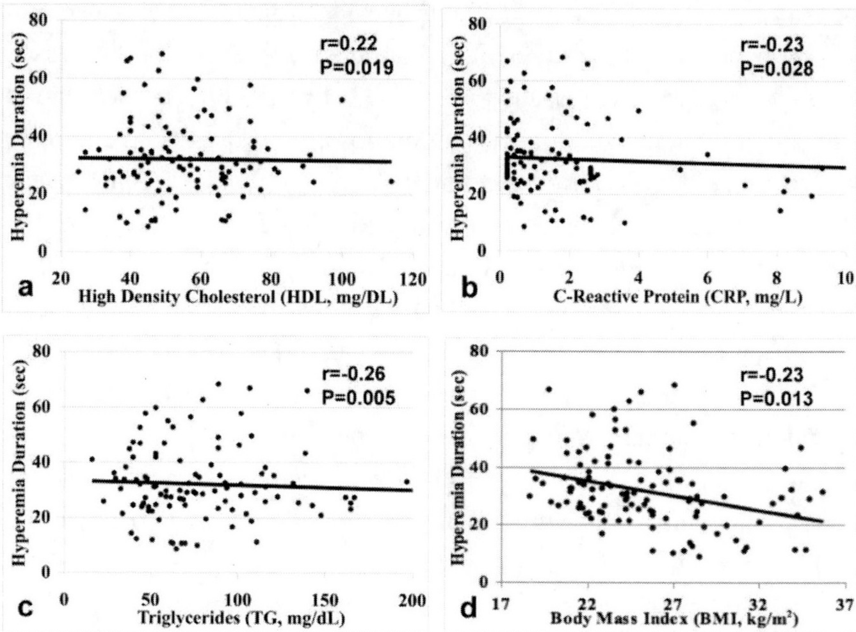

Figure 1. Significant correlations between MRI vascular reactivity metric - hyperemia duration or forward flow time (T_{ff}), and biomarker indices (|r| > 0.2, P < 0.05).

Our longitudinal analysis showed that at 18-month follow-up time, strong correlations between MRI parameters and multiple cardiovascular factors were present in especially elderly participants and smokers. An example of significant correlations between longitudinal MRI vascular reactivity parameter- hyperemia duration or forward flow time (Tff) that mimics ischemia condition after cuff release and indicates vascular reactivity time, and cardiovascular biomarkers including high-density cholesterol (HDL) level (r = 0.22, 0.019), C-reactive protein (CRP) (r = -0.23, P < 0.0001), triglycerides (TG) (r = -0.26, P = 0.005) as well as body mass index (BMI) (r = -

0.23, P = 0.013) is given in Figure 1. Moreover, significant correlations between cardiovascular factors at initial visit including SBP and smoking pack years, and MRI parameters at 18-month follow-ups indicated that these cardiovascular risk factors (e.g., blood pressure and smoking severity) could cause endothelial dysfunction such as arterial stiffness with age and in smokers.

In summary, we reported longitudinal neuroimaging changes of both structural and functional connectivity in regions that were similar to those demonstrating cross-sectional effects of age; for instance decreased functional connectivity in default mode network but increased connectivity in anti-correlated dorso-attentional network together with prominent structural connectivity and integrity deterioration. Furthermore, these brain changes were highly correlated with neurocognitive dysfunction, especially in the domains of memory, cognitive flexibility, visual perception and attention, and executive function. The genetic influence such as APOE genotypic signatures of FA and functional connectivity suggested possible tight associations between myelin/neuronal activation and APOE gene, indicating different roles of APOE alleles on brain structural conductivity, demyelination and neuroplasticity. We had also found significantly worsening of microvascular reactivity and arterial stiffness with age and in smokers, at both central nervous and peripheral systems at both initial and 18-month follow-up visits. There were variable degrees of longitudinal changes of higher tau deposition, amyloid accumulation and FDG hypometabolism with age. High sensitivity and specificity of the applied imaging metrics suggested detectable pathological, structural and functional brain changes at both molecular and macroscopic levels. Finally, the significant baseline and longitudinal correlations between MRI parameters and cardiovascular risk factors in addition to neurocognitive function could provide distinct and confirmative evidences as well as treatment guidance relating to the aging-related diseases such as dementia, cardiac disease, atherosclerosis, stroke, hypertension and diabetes.

REFERENCES

[1] Abner EL, Nelson PT, Schimtt FA, Diabetes is associated with cerebrovascular but not Alzheimer's disease neuropathology, *Alzheimer's & Dementia*, 2016; 12: 882-889.

[2] Aguilar-Salinas C.A., Rojas R., Gó mez-Pe rez F.J., Valles V., Ríos-Torres J.M., Franco A., Olaiz G., Rull J.A., Sepulveda J., Analysis of the agreement between the World Health Organization criteria and the National Cholesterol Education Program-III definition of the metabolic syndrome: results from a population-based survey, *Diabetes Care*, 2003;26:1635.

[3] Alberti K.G., Zimmet P.Z., Definition, diagnosis and classification of diabetes mellitus and its complications. Part 1: diagnosis and classification of diabetes mellitus provisional report of a WHO consultation, *Diabet. Med.*, 1998; 15:539 –553.

[4] American Psychiatric Association (APA), *Diagnostic and Statistical Manual of Mental Disorders*, DSM-IV, 1994.

[5] Bales CW, Locher JL, Saltzman E, *Handbook of Clinical Nutrition and Aging*, Humana Press, 2015.

[6] Baltes PB, Lindenberger U. Emergence of a powerful connection between sensory and cognitive functions across the adult life span: A new window to the study of cognitive aging? *Psychology and Aging*, 1997; 12:12–21.

[7] Bender AR and Raz N, Normal-appearing cerebral white matter in healthy adults: mean change over 2 years and individual differences in change, *Neurobiology of aging*, 2015; 36:1834-1848.

[8] Boecker H, Hillman CH, Scheef L, Strüder HK, Functional Neuroimaging in Exercise and Sport Sciences, Springer, 2012.

[9] Bonomini F, Fabrizio L, Mezzani RR, Metabolic Syndrome, Aging and Involvement of Oxidative Stress, *Aging and Disease*, 2015; 6(2):109-120.

[10] Churilla JR, Fitzhugh EC, Thompson DL, The metabolic syndrome: how definition impacts the prevalence and risk among U.S. adults, NHANES 1999 –2004. *Metab Syndr Relat Disord*, 2007; 5:331–342.

[11] Clark LR, Koscik RL, Allison SL, et al., Hypertension and obesity moderate the relationship between β-amyloid and cognitive decline in midlife, *Alzheimer's & Dementia*, 2018; 1-10.

[12] Cohen G, Research on creativity and aging: The positive impact of the arts on health and illness, *Generations*, 2006; 30: 7–15.

[13] Craft S and Christen Y, *Diabetes, Insulin and Alzheimer's Disease*. Springer, 2009.

[14] de la Torre JC, *Alzheimer's Turning Point: A Vascular Approach to Clinical Prevention*, Springer, 2016.

[15] Everitt AV, Couteur D.G, Rattan SIS, de Cabo R, *Calorie Restriction, Aging and Longevity*, Springer, 2010.

[16] Ford E.S., Giles W.H., Dietz W.H., Prevalence of the metabolic syndrome among US adults: findings from the third National Health and Nutrition Examination Survey, *JAMA*, 2002; 287:356 –359.

[17] Ford ES, Giles WH, Mokdad AH, Increasing prevalence of the metabolic syndrome among U.S. adults, *Diabetes Care*, 2004; 27:2444 –2449.

[18] Fratiglioni L, Paillard-Borg S, & Winblad B. An active and socially integrated lifestyle in late life might protect against dementia, *Lancet. Neurology*, 2004; 3:343.

[19] Grundy SM, Brewer HB Jr, Cleeman JI, Smith SC Jr, Lenfant C, American Heart Association, National Heart, Lung, and Blood Institute. Definition of metabolic syndrome: report of the National Heart, Lung, and Blood Institute/American Heart Association conference on scientific issues related to definition. *Circulation*, 2004; 109: 433– 438.

[20] Gullette MM, *Aged by Culture*, University of Chicago Press, 2004.

[21] Jack CR, Wiste HJ, Weigand SD, et al., Age-specific population frequencies of cerebral β-amyloidosis and neurodegeneration among people with normal cognitive function aged 50–89 years: a cross-sectional study, *Lancet Neurol* 2014; 13: 997–1005.

[22] Kemppainen J., Aalto S., Fujimoto T., Kalliokoski K.K., Langsjo J., Oikonen V., Rinne J., Nuutila P., Knuuti J., High intensity exercise decreases global brain glucose uptake in humans, *J Physiol.*, 2005; 568:323–332.

[23] Langham MC, Zhou Y, Chirico EN, Magland JF, Sehgal CM, Englund EK, Mohler III RE, Guo W, Barhoum S, Wehrli FW, "Effects of Age and Smoking on Endothelial Function Assessed by Quantitative MRI and Ultrasound in the Peripheral and Central Vasculature," *Journal of Cardiovascular Magnetic Resonance*, 2015; 17 (1):19.

[24] Lefevre M, Redman LM, Heilbronn LK, Smith JV, Martin CK, Rood JC, Greenway FL, Williamson DA, Smith SR and Ravussin E, Pennington CALERIE team, Calorie restriction alone and with exercise improves CVD risk in healthy non-obese individuals. *Atherosclerosis*, 2009; 203: 206–213.

[25] Lewis JS and Keshari KR, *Imaging and Metabolism*, Springer, 2018.

[26] Lindauer M, *Aging, creativity and art: A positive perspective on late-life development*. Springer Science & Business Media, 2003.

[27] Menec VH, The relation between everyday activities and successful aging: A 6-year longitudinal study. *The Journals of Gerontology – Series B, Psychological Sciences and Social Sciences*, 2003; 58:S74.

[28] Morley JE, The Metabolic Syndrome and Aging, *Journal of Gerontology: Medical Science*, 2004; 59(2):139–142.

[29] Mozumdar A and Liguori G, Persistent Increase of Prevalence of Metabolic Syndrome Among US Adults: NHANES III to NHANES 1999–2006, 2011; *Diabetes Care*, 34: 216–219.

[30] Raz N, and Rodigue KM, Differential aging of the brain: Patterns, cognitive correlates and modifiers. *Neurosci. Beh. Reviews*, 2006; 30: 730–748.

[31] Raz N, Lindenberger U, Rodrigue KM, Kennedy KM, Head D, Williamson A, Acker JD, Regional brain changes in aging healthy adults: General trends, individual differences, and modifiers, *Cer. Cortex*, 2005; 15:1676–1689.

[32] Ravussin E., Redman L.M., Caloric restriction and longevity, *Journ Annu Diabetol Hotel Dieu*, 2007;111-125.

[33] Redman LM, Heilbronn LK, Martin CK, de Jonge L, Williamson DA, Delany JP, Ravussin E and Pennington CALERIE Team, Metabolic and behavioral compensations in response to caloric restriction, implications for the maintenance of weight loss, *PLoS One* 2009; 4: e4377.

[34] Redman LM, Martin CK, Williamson DA and Ravussin E, Effect of caloric restriction in non-obese humans on physiological, psychological and behavioral outcomes, *Physiol Behav*, 2008; 94: 643–648.

[35] Rizzo M, Anderson S, Fritzsch B, *The Wiley Handbook on the Aging Mind and Brain*, John Wiley & Sons Ltd, 2018.

[36] Sohal R.S., Weindruch R., Oxidative stress, caloric restriction, and aging, *Science*, 1996; 273(5271):59-63. 2018.

[37] Speakman JR, Talbot DA, Selman C, Snart S, Mclaren JS, Redman P, Krol E, Jackson DM, Johnson MS and Brand MD, Uncoupled and surviving: individual mice with high metabolism have greater mitochondrial uncoupling and live longer, *Ageing Cell*, 2004; 3:87–95.

[38] Stern Y, Cognitive reserve, *Neuropsychologia*, 2009; 47: 2015–2018.

[39] Thakur MK and Rattan SIS, *Brain Aging and Therapeutic Interventions*, Springer, 2012.

[40] Toledo JB, Arnold M, Kastenmuller G, Metabolic network failures in Alzheimer's disease: A biochemical road map, *Alzheimer's & Dementia*, 2017; 13: 965-984.

[41] Ugurbil K, Berliner L, Uludag K, *FMRI: From Nuclear Spins to Brain Functions*, Springer, 2015.

[42] Weiner MW, Veitch DP, Aisen PS, et al., Recent publications from the Alzheimer's Disease Neuroimaging Initiative: Reviewing progress toward improved AD clinical trials, *Alzheimer's & Dementia*, 2017; 13: e1-e85.

[43] World Health Organization, *Definition, diagnosis and classification of diabetes mellitus and its complications: Report of a WHO Consultation.* Part 1: diagnosis and classification of diabetes mellitus, 1999.

[44] Zhao Q, Chen X and Zhou Y, Quantitative multimodal multiparametric imaging in Alzheimer's disease, *Brain Informatics*, 2016; 3:29–37.

[45] Zhou Y, book, *Functional Neuroimaging with Multiple Modalities: Principles, Device and Applications*, Nova Science Publishers, 2016.

[46] Zhou Y, book chapter, Cerebral Blood Flow Mediated Rapid Vascular Reactivity Mapping and Effects of Age and Smoking, *Horizons in Neuroscience Research*, Nova Science Publishers, 2017, Volume. 31: 57-91.

[47] Zhou Y, book, *Functional Neuroimaging Methods and Frontiers*. Nova Publishers, 2018.

About the Author

Yongxia Zhou

University of Southern California, Los Angeles, CA

Columbia University, New York, NY

Yongxia Zhou is a medical imaging scientist, specialized in MRI neuroimaging and neurosciences applications. She had completed my PhD from University of Southern California in Biomedical imaging in 2004 and had been trained and worked as neuroimaging scientists in several prestigious institutes including Columbia University, New York University and University of Pennsylvania and NIH. Her research focuses on multi-modal neuroimaging including using MRI/PET and EEG instrumentation as well as the integration of these multi-modal to make the best usage of each modality and to help interpreting underlying co-existing pathophysiological for better disease diagnosis and treatment. Her specific interests in MRI technology include brain mapping of blood flow, oxygen saturation and extraction fraction and metabolism as well as vascular reactivity assessment with fMRI activity/connectivity and arterial spin labeling (ASL)-based blood flow measures. She had published several books and book chapters, about 100 papers and abstracts in well known international journals and conferences. She has been serving as several journal and international conference reviewers including JMRI, JCBFM, HBM, AJNR, Plos One, ISMRM and ICAD.

INDEX

B

C

D

E

F

G

H

I

K

L

M

N

O

P

Q

R

S

T

U

V

W

Y